# ACTIVITY CARE PLANS
# FOR
# LONG TERM CARE FACILITIES

## (or, if you didn't write it down, it wasn't done!)

## FOURTH EDITION

Pamela Sander, TRS/TXC

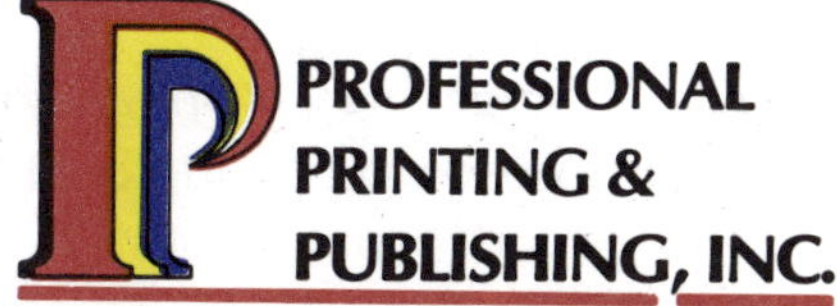

PROFESSIONAL
PRINTING &
PUBLISHING, INC.

P.O. Box 5758 · Bossier City, LA 71171-5758
318-746-6880 · 1-800-551-8783 · FAX 318-746-6995
Web Site: http://www.ppandp.com
E-mail: order@ppandp.com

FOURTH EDITION 1999

THIRD EDITION 1992
Five Printings

SECOND EDITION 1988
Seven Printings

FIRST EDITION 1984
Five Printings


ISBN 1-877735-05-1


Professional Printing & Publishing, Inc.
P.O. Box 5758
Bossier City, LA 71171-5758
318/746-6880
WATS 1-800/551-8783 - FAX 318/746-6995
Web Site: http://www.ppandp.com
E-mail: order@ppandp.com

For my great aunt, Ada DePass Patterson, who taught me the importance of "writing it down"; for Vincent Tassin, LPT, who taught me "Care planning can be fun"; for Eddie, the guiding light in my life; for Nolan S. who helped me to see the importance of sharing what I know; for all the Activity Directors and residents in those long term care facilities where I consult, who continue to teach me daily… I offer you this book, the sum total of my care plan knowledge today. This is just a beginning…

# About the Author

Pamela Sander is a therapeutic recreation specialist with over thirty years experience in health care, specializing since 1976 in the field of long term care activity programs.  Pam, as she prefers to be called is a graduate of Louisiana State University, 1968, with postgraduate studies at LSU, Tulane, and University of New Orleans.  Since moving from Louisiana to Texas in 1978, Pam has worked as a consultant to nursing homes, hospital based skilled nursing units, and assisted living centers activity programs.  She has also taught both the 90-hour Basic Education and the 90-hour Advanced Management courses for long term care activity personnel; and, has provided numerous continuing education workshops for activity and other long term care personnel in Texas, throughout the southern states, in the mid-west, and on the east coast of the United States. Pam's health care experience also includes physical rehabilitation, psychosocial rehabilitation and leisure counseling.  She began her career in long term care at a 200-bed facility in New Orleans as Director of Activity Therapy.

Pam's books include ***Care Plans That Work with the MDS 2.0, Policies and Procedures for Activity Programs and Volunteer Services,*** and ***Wake Up! A Sensory Stimulation Program for Nursing Home Residents.***

Pam is certified in Texas with the Consortium for Therapeutic Recreation/Activities Certification and is an active member of the Texas Recreation and Parks Society, Therapeutic Recreation Branch. Pam is also currently an ad hoc faculty member with Austin Community College after serving seventeen years as ad hoc faculty with North Harris College, Houston.

Ms. Sander, originally from New Orleans, Louisiana, is currently residing in Austin, Texas.

# Forward

Over the last thirty years, I have taught and/or worked with over (500) five hundred new Activity Directors.  Always, in every class or when orienting a new Activity Director the same questions surface.  Sometimes it takes several weeks — at other times the questions are asked on the first day:

> "If I do all the paper work required when will I have time to work with my residents?"

> "Why are care plans so important?"

> "How can I be expected to do all this writing, and do everything else I have to do?"

> etc. etc. etc.

Composition of the questions may vary, but the same frustration runs throughout because of the amount of paperwork required in running an activity program in a nursing facility and the importance placed on it.  Almost always the dread of doing the writing consumes more time than the actual recording of the information itself.  Some are fearful of what others will think about what they write, or "how" they write what is recorded.  Others are concerned about the fact that the health care plan is part of the medical record and as such could be subpoenaed in a court of law.  While still others don't quite know how to express what they want to say, or what they feel should be said.

Regardless, what generally occurs next is a "falling behind" in the schedule.  The resident assessments and health care plans go "undone" for too long.  The survey team comes into the facility for a review, and deficiencies are cited.  Then, sometimes more often than many would be willing to admit, a really good activity director loses her job.  A new person is hired, must begin by playing "documentation catchup", and the cycle continues.

My purpose in writing this text is to help break this cycle, to provide instruction to new Activity Directors and to offer a frame of reference that will in some way remotivate those of you who have been "in the business" for a period of time. To that end, I have divided this text into three major sections:  (1) How to Write a Care Plan, (2) Sample Problems/Needs, Short Term Goals, and Approaches, (3) Glossary of Activities and Terms used in the text.

Keep in mind, when using the information in this book, that this is just a place to begin.  This book is in no way the "complete text of health care plans."  There is not enough paper to document a book such as that.  For just as each of you is different, so is every resident in your nursing facility different with different needs, wants, quirks, and desires. Therefore, each health care plan is, or should be, different. Do not limit yourself to the language used here; instead use my language here as a "primer," then go forward to develop your own.

Pamela Sander, TRS/TXC

# Table of Contents

# SECTION I
## How To Write A Care Plan



# SECTION II
## Sample Problems/Needs, Short Term Goals, And Approaches

# SECTION III

## Glossary of Activities and Terms

# SECTION I

## How To Write A Care Plan

# How To Write An Activity Health Care Plan

Ever since 1974, when health care plans were first required by the federal regulations for facilities participating in the Medicaid and/or Medicare program, problems related to health-care planning have been an enigma for most activity personnel.  "Care Planning" is a chore dreaded by many usually because of one basic fear we all share — fear of the unknown.  Federal regulations and state standards tell us what is required, but do not offer any guidelines as to how these requirements are to be achieved.  This fear is compounded by the volume of care plans to be written and rewritten.  Thus one can easily become "overwhelmed" and "consumed" by the care plan process.

With the implementation of the OBRA regulations in 1989 and the current update of those rules in 1990, 1993, 1995, and 1999, the comprehensive assessment and overall plan of care has taken an even greater significance.  OBRA requires the use of the HCFA form for comprehensive assessment of the resident and a plan of care developed from this assessment.  For the first time in the history of the Medicare and Medicaid programs, the federal government is requiring use of a specific form in all Title 18 and Title 19 participating facilities in this country — the Minimum Data Set, Version 2.0 or the MDS[1] as it is referred to by health-care professionals.  This MDS is just that, a minimal assessment of the resident.  Facilities are not required to use any one care plan form; however, regulations require that whatever format is chosen, that it be comprehensive and interdisciplinary, i.e., that all the residents' problems (needs) be addressed and

---

[1] MDS 2.0 — this is the second or third generation version of the MDS, depending on which state the reader lives.  The original MDS put in use in 1990 was altered into several "MDS+" forms in use by test pilot states.  Then in 1995 all the MDS forms were converged into this MDS 2.0.  This last 2.0 form is used universally across the country and has become the basis for the new (1999) survey process using the MDS as a means of determining the "Quality Indicators" for the survey teams' focus.  HCFA allows each state to individualize the form by including a state-developed "Section S," if the state desires.

that anyone and everyone who has responsibilities for providing "care" for the resident have input into this plan.

The care plan process (which includes the initial comprehensive assessment) utilized by facility staff now is the most important document in the resident's medical record.  Since 1986 the survey process mandated by the feds has focused on resident care and outcome of this care.  With OBRA the surveyors are looking even closer still at the effects of care delivered.  The OBRA surveyors are interviewing residents, asking questions regarding the resident's point of view of care delivered as well as assessing for themselves "what" is being done and "why" it is being done.  After making their own detailed assessment the surveyors then pull the resident's current records and review to determine whether or not facility staff have identified the same problem/need areas and what is being done by facility staff and/or others to help residents satisfy these problems and/ or needs.  The central documents reviewed in this process are the MDS, subsequent additional assessments and the comprehensive care plan.  These documents establish "what" care is given, "why" this care is given, "how often" and "when", as well as by "whom".

With the new survey process (1999) and the use of transmitted MDS assessments, the surveyors now have access to residents' MDS assessments in their field offices.  Part of the advanced preparation for the new annual surveys is to review the most recent MDS transmitted on each resident, deduct information regarding the Quality Indicators from these MDS assessments, select the group of residents who will be identified for in-depth survey review, and plan the overall focus of the survey.  All of this advanced work, including review of each facility's OSCAR report, occurs before the survey teams leave their offices to begin a survey in the chosen facility.

There are a variety of activity assessment forms and comprehensive care plan forms available for use.  Some are helpful in documenting what is required, but more often some just add to the confusion because of the repetition of information and overlap of their use.

Unfortunately one simple fact is often overlooked amid the variety of forms available.  "All health care plans have six basic components," regardless of the form used.  These are:

(1)   data collection and assessment

(2)   statements of problems and/or needs

(3)   long term goals

(4)   short term goals (or objectives)

(5)   approaches (or plans)

(6)   reassessment (new data collection) and update

In the following pages, I shall attempt to define the above terms and provide insight as to how one can best record a thorough, informative activity health care plan; i.e. how to write a good activity care plan. Remember, as an old professor of mine use to say, if you don't have time to do it RIGHT now, when will you have the time to do it OVER...

## (1)  Data Collection and Assessment

No care plan can be written until the Activity Director knows the resident.  The only way is to begin by collecting data or information about the resident's past as well as his/her present.  In order to do this it is important to use a combination of observation and interviewing of the resident, the family, and the environment from which the resident hails.  You will want to familiarize yourself with pertinent medical and non-medical history including such information as sex, age, birthdate, marital status, current family situation, place of birth, religion, living arrangements or situation before admission to the nursing facility, where childhood was spent, how many siblings and birth order of resident, occupation, lifetime interests, hobbies, skills, leisure skills, etc., as well as health information both current and past. You can obtain this data through conversation with the resident and any family or friends who may visit.  Ideally, this initial data should be collected at the time of admission, through use of an admission interview with the resident and his/her family present at admission. Use of an interest checklist may be helpful.

Remember, it is your responsibility as Activity Director to impress on others — family, residents, and other staff members — the importance of your becoming involved from the very beginning so that you can assist the new resident into adapting to life in the nursing facility.  If you sit back and wait to be asked to become involved, then you might find yourself collecting dust...

Keep this admission interview brief and to the point; allow a certain amount of time and stick to it.  Also, and most importantly, make arrangements for future interview time to obtain more information needed.  Explain to the family your reasons for requesting this information, i.e. "I want to help your mother adjust to living here and to introduce her to other residents with similar interests."

During this initial interview and subsequent interviews observe how the resident and his/her family interact.  Make particular notice of whether the family and resident seem comfortable with each other. Does the resident speak for himself/herself or does the family member seem to take control?  Is there a presence of tension and/or emotion? or, a lack of emotion?  Was the resident involved in making the decision about living in a nursing facility? or, did the family..., the doctor..., or someone else make this decision? Does the family visit and/or call about the resident?  When the family and the resident are together is there any physical contact?  Does this contact seem forced?... or, is there much obvious affection shown toward each other?  Which family members seem to be in control?  Who takes responsibility for answering your inquiries? Be observant! Record your observations as soon after the interview as possible, while they are still fresh in your mind.  Record only behavior observed so as not to influence your notes with your own personal feelings.

Observe how the resident interacts with other residents in the facility. Has the resident begun any steps toward friendship with his/her roommate and/or neighbor? Does the resident initiate conversation? ...respond to conversational attempts of others? ...get involved in conversation? ...only respond with nods of head, grunts, one word answers? Is the resident able to communicate? If not, why not? Is the communication verbal or non-verbal?

What about group situations? Since admission, has the resident expressed or shown any interest in the variety of programs offered? Has the resident attended any activities? When in a group situation does the resident stay on the fringe of the group, observing? ...actively participate in whatever is occurring? ...or refuse to become involved at all?

How does the resident spend his/her day? Does he/she sit in room alone? ...watch TV - in room, or in community television room? Does he/she read? ...regular or large print books? What kind of reading material appeals to the resident? How does the resident seek attention from others?...cries?...grunts?...yells or screams? What is the resident's orientation to self and surroundings? Is resident able to feed self?...dress self? Is resident able to find items in his/her room? When out of room, is resident able to locate dining room?...TV room?...living room?...own room? Is the resident able to tell time?...read a calendar? Does the resident recognize others?... remember names of others? What about memory?

How does the resident ambulate? Does he/she walk with a walker?...independent?...use a wheelchair?...gerichair?...bedfast? If the resident uses a wheelchair, does he/she know how to make the wheels turn?...use both hands to turn wheels? Does he/she need help getting around the nursing facility?

Are there any special medical or nutritional needs that would affect the resident's involvement in the activity program? What about allergies? Is the resident able to see?...hear?...speak? Is the resident particularly sensitive to heat?...cold?...loud noises?

What about behavior? Has the resident displayed any overt behavior since admission? The questions go on, and on.

These are basic questions for which you should seek answers in assessing a resident's activity needs. They are in no way all inclusive, but should be used as a springboard to better evaluate the resident. In documenting the activity assessment it is important to remember that the opinions or judgments of you, the Activity Director, are not significant. What is significant is the observed behavior which gave you the answers to these and other such questions. Obviously, this information cannot be gathered through a few brief interviews. Instead, you should take time in carefully evaluating the resident through multiple interviews and observation of the resident in a variety of situations over several days. Be assured that initial assessments are apt to change both with time and as you and the resident become more familiar with each other.

Record the required information on the MDS, Section I. Record the additional data collected on your chosen Activity Assessment form. Whatever form you chose to use to record this initial data, be sure your form allows enough space to be thorough. I prefer a form which lists the different areas covered in the aforementioned questions and then provides me with a place to write a "word picture" of the resident, thus tying all the data together into a narrative. The narrative, if properly written, will then help set up and support the needs, goals, and approaches for the completion of the first care plan. See the sample care plan at the back of this section.

## (2)  Statement of Problems and/or Needs

For the purpose of this text, problems will be defined as a situation or condition that causes or creates, or may cause or create distress for the resident; or interferes with the resident's adjustment or involvement with others. A need is a condition which requires some sort of supply and/or relief. Identification of needs is very important. Not all residents have problems in the area of activities, but all have needs. Needs that are not identified and subsequently not met become problems.

In considering what the resident's problems and/or needs may be, the Activity Director should give thought to the "pluses" (positive qualities of the resident) as well as "minuses." It is important to realize that the resident is a "total person" with needs, wants, habits, likes, dislikes, as well as "problems." It is so very easy to get caught up in the negative and totally overlook the whole person in the process. All of our residents have needs and/or problems; otherwise they would not be living in the nursing facility. In order to help the resident adapt to life in your home, you should build from his/her strengths and in so doing help the resident to compensate for, adjust to, or overcome the weaknesses that interfere with this process.

If your initial assessment is thorough, the problems and/or needs will just pop out at you. Simply look for those areas that are a cause of distress for the resident or that interfere with the resident's ability to make the most of his life in your facility. Make a list of the resident's strengths and weaknesses. Look at the weaknesses and make some determination as to which areas to help the resident "work on" first. Discuss this with the resident. After all, if the resident does not agree there is a problem and/or a need for change, then you will be defeating your own purpose and subsequently setting unrealistic goals. If "it," whatever you have outlined "it" to be, is not a problem for the resident, is "it" then a problem? This is a question that has no pat answer. You must use your own common sense and past experience as a guideline. It may well be that the first area you are called on to give assistance to is the resident's attitude regarding his/her ability and/or willingness to affect change in himself/herself.

In those situations where the resident is unable to give input into his/her care plan, you will want to "tackle" the "weaknesses" that interfere with the resident's ability to maintain a sense of security about himself/herself and his/her new home, i.e. help him to adjust to the physical layout of the home, feel a sense of trust toward those who work with him/her, maintain some sort of comfort in the life-style limited by his/her physical being and/or provide a few moments of pleasure. For sample problems see the case study at the end of this section and the sample in Section II.

## (3) Long Term Goals

A long term goal is an overall statement of where the resident could be or what the resident will achieve over a period of time, usually a year or more. The statements are general in nature and may vary from individual to individual.

Sample long term goals may include:

1.   Will be able to talk with others comfortably.

2.   Will participate actively in activities of the nursing facility.

3.   Will adjust to life in nursing facility.

4.   Will make friends in the nursing facility.

5.   Will live in comfort and maintain personal dignity.

6.   Will be discharged back home.

     etc.  etc.  etc.

For an example of the use of a long term goal in practical application, see the sample case study health care plan at the end of this section and the chart illustrating short term goals as steps to achieve the overall long term goal.

Some facilities prefer that all staff work toward the same overall long term goal. This makes sense. If this is the policy of your nursing facility, add your input to the long term goal. For example: "Mr. Smith will adjust to life in the nursing facility, accept the care given him, be adequately nourished and will make friends with other residents of similar interests."

## (4)  Short Term Goals

If long term goals can be considered as the major plateaus one reaches on the mountain-side, then short term goals are the individual steps one takes to reach each plateau.  For example:

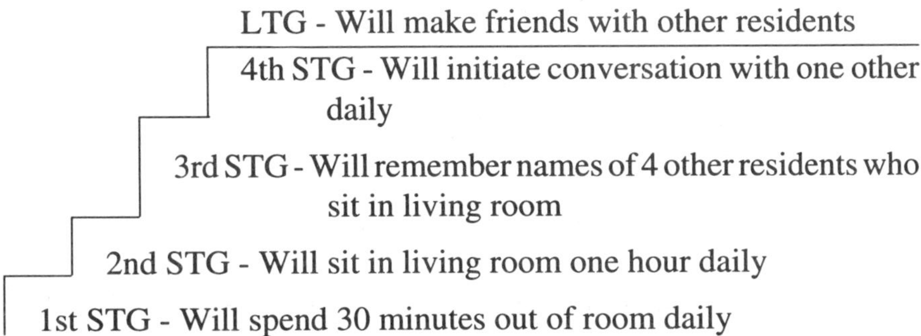


Short term goals are statements of action, on the part of the resident, that are behaviorally observable and can be measured over time.  Key words are "Resident will…(perform some action) _______ (number of times) by __________ (date)."  In writing short term goals, use action words such as: walk, talk, sit, remember, respond, write, draw, eat, participate, attend, touch, identify, observe, discuss, etc.  Precede these action words with "resident will…" then include how many times, and/or when, and/or where followed by the date that this will be accomplished; then, Voila! You have written a short term goal.  Example: "Resident will talk (action word) with three others (number) in the living room (where) daily (when) by the next update (date).

When goal setting, involve the resident as much as possible.  It just makes good sense to help your residents to set their own goals.  In that way, you have some sort of assurance that the resident will work toward the achievement of these goals.  Also, keep the goals realistic.  Short term goals that have not been achieved after three months or so under close inspection may be too big a step to take at one shot.  Using your knowledge of the resident's strengths (a good assessment), set goals that are achievable and build from there.  Sample short term goals are located in Section II of this book as well as in the sample case study at the end of this section.

## (5)  Approaches

Approaches are the statements of actions that others will take to help the resident achieve the stated short term goal.  Approaches should be laid out in such a way so that anyone who reads the care plan will be able to understand "who" will be doing "what" to help the resident overcome his/her problems and/or satiate his/her needs.  The person performing the action should be identified.

Examples:

1.   All staff should use the resident's name frequently.

2.   Volunteer will visit and talk with resident about bird feeders.

3.   Activity Director and/or assistant will escort resident to bingo.

4.   Activity Director will invite resident to religious services.

For more examples, see Section II of this book and the sample case study at the end of this section.


## (6)  Reassessment and Update (the process begins again)

The Activity Care Plan is reassessed and updated as often as is necessary or at least once a quarter (every 90 days).  While the reassessment information is not always as lengthy as the initial assessment, it should be just as thorough.  Reassessment information should include:

(1)  Direct reference to the achievement or lack of achievement of short term goals.

(2)  Information regarding the effectiveness of the stated approaches.

(3)  Activity participation, which ones, to what extent, how involved.

(4)  Behavior since last assessment.

(5)  Interaction with other residents, family, visitors, volunteers, staff, etc.

(6)  General statements of how resident spends his day.

(7)  Degree of involvement on the part of the resident in setting new goals and updating of the health care plan.

Assessment and reassessment is an on-going never ending process. Upon completion of the reassessment narrative, it is time now to set new goals and formulate approaches.  Problems and/or needs that have been resolved should be identified as such, and new needs recorded.  And so it goes...

## Why Is Care Planning So Important?

It doesn't matter how many times you may have involved "Mr. Jones" in a handicraft project or how frequently "Mr. Smith" goes to exercise class, if there is no written record, then theoretically the activity did not exist.  We are living in an age of lawsuits.  Just because we, as Activity Directors, are not always directly involved in the physical aspect of medical care does not mean we could not be held as a responsible party should the facility be liable.  If "Mrs. Jones" family should decide that the care she receives is not meeting her needs then her family may institute plans to transfer her to another facility or worse, take judiciary action.  If there is no written record of "Mrs. Jones" participation or lack of participation and why, then you as Activity Director are at fault.  Surely your time is more valuable to your residents in the facility than sitting in a courtroom or some lawyer's office.

Health Care Plans are direct proof of your effectiveness as a recreator. They become invaluable in the acquisition of more volunteers, raises in pay, the purchase of new equipment, etc. Statistics formulated from your health care plans on the number of people who may be using a dilapidated ping-pong table can certainly be an asset in requisitioning a new one.  Also in participating in care planning with other members of the health care team you are sharing your policies, procedures, and philosophies so that other staff better understand the importance of their support in the activity process.  Care planning sessions are an informative time to exchange and share information about resident behavior.  "Mrs. Jones" may not be attending a much loved sewing session in the afternoon because she is having lunch with "Mr. Smith" who ridicules "women who sew."  Without the give and take of communication which care plan sessions provide, it would be difficult, if not impossible to achieve the continuity of total staff care.  In formulating your care plans you need feedback from the rest of the facility staff, as well as the resident.  This feedback assists you in program planning, evaluation, and reevaluation.  Care plans are a meaningful aid in determining the effectiveness of your activity program.

Let yourself feel good when charting or participating in care planning on a particularly successful resident.  If you don't toot your own horn, who will?

# Sample Case Study

## Activity Health Care Plan

**Assessment:** (begun on the first day of admission and completed within the first 14 days)

Resident, Mrs. Agnes Jones, is an 87 year w/f, admitted 8/14/99, from home by her daughter, Mrs. Alma Smith. Resident has an admission diagnosis of arthritis, Diabetes Mellitus, Parkinson's Syndrome, and a history of a stroke in 1986. Resident was born in Columbus, Ohio, August 22, 1913; the oldest of six children, three are currently residing in Texas. At the age of fourteen, Mrs. Jones and her family moved to Houston, where a year later resident met and married Allen W. Jones. Mr. and Mrs. Jones raised four children, two by their marriage, and two from a previous marriage of Mr. Jones. The Jones lived together in the same house in the Montrose area of Houston until Mr. Jones' death in 1991. At that time Mrs. Jones went to live with her youngest daughter, Mrs. Alma Smith. Mrs. Jones completed eight years of schooling in Ohio, then worked as a clerk in the family dry-goods store in Houston until she married Mr. Jones in 1928. At that time Mrs. Jones retired to help raise Mr. Jones' two children and have two more of her own, the first in 1935 and the second, Mrs. Smith, in 1938.

Mrs. Jones had a minor stroke in 1986, which did not seem to leave any residual effects, but when Mr. Jones died in 1991, both mother and daughter decided it would be better for Mrs. Jones to live with Mrs. Smith's family. There are two grown children in this branch of Mrs. Jones' family; three grandchildren from her first born child, and a total of four from the two children of Mr. Jones. All but two of the grandchildren live away from Houston. Mrs. Jones keeps in touch with these grandchildren through telephone conversations, cards, and letters.

Mrs. Jones is currently confined to a wheelchair because of her severe, crippling arthritis. She is able to ambulate herself around in the nursing facility in the wheelchair without assistance, but needs help when outside of the building.  She is independent in eating when using a special built-up spoon for that purpose; needs assistance in dressing and bathing.  She is currently taking medications for her arthritis and Parkinson's.  Her diabetes is controlled by a regular diet with no concentrated sugars.  Mrs. Jones has no problems with her diet, as she says, "I've been on it for a number of years…since I turned sixty."

## SECTION N.  ACTIVITY PURSUIT PATTERNS

| 1. | **Time Awake** <br> 10B only if BOTH N1a = ✓ and N2 =0 | (Check appropriate time period over last 7 days) <br> Resident awake all or most of time (i.e., naps no more than one hour per time period) in the: <br><br> Morning **10B** — a. ✓ — Evening — c. ✓ <br> Afternoon — b. ✓ — *NONE OF ABOVE* — d. |
|---|---|---|

### (IF RESIDENT IS COMATOSE, SKIP TO SECTION O)

| 2. | **AVERAGE TIME INVOLVED IN ACTIVITIES** | (When awake and not receiving treatments or ADL care) <br><br> 0. Most — more than 2/3 of time **10B**    2. Little — less than 1/3 of time **10A** <br> 1. Some — from 1/3 to 2/3 of time    3. None **10A**    **1** |
|---|---|---|
| 3. | **PREFERRED ACTIVITY SETTINGS** | (*Check all settings* in which activities are *preferred*) <br><br> Own room — a. <br> Day / activity room — b. ✓    Outside facility — d. <br> Inside NH/off unit — c. ✓    *NONE OF ABOVE* — e. |
| 4. | **GENERAL ACTIVITY PREFER-ENCES** <br> (Adapted to resident's current abilities) | (*Check all PREFERENCES* whether or not activity is currently available to resident) <br><br> Cards/other games — a.    Trips/shopping — g. <br> Crafts/arts — b. ✓    Walking/wheeling outdoors — h. ✓ <br> Exercise/sports — c. ✓    Watching TV — i. ✓ <br> Music — d.    Gardening or plants — j. <br> Reading/writing — e. ✓    Talking or conversing — k. ✓ <br> Spiritual/religious activities — f. ✓    Helping others — l. <br>    *NONE OF ABOVE* — m. |
| 5. | **PREFERS CHANGE IN DAILY ROUTINE** | Code for resident preferences in daily routines <br> 0. No change    1. Slight change    2. Major change <br><br> a. Type of activities in which resident is currently involved 1 or 2 = **10A**    **0** <br> b. Extent of resident involvement in activity 1 or 2 = **10A**    **0** |

(Note:  The information recorded in Section N, Activity Pursuit Patterns, of the MDS 2.0 does not indicate any problems have been triggered or identified.  Thus the importance of a more thorough activity assessment becomes paramount as is evident in this continuing narrative assessment of Mrs. Jones.)

Since admission, Mrs. Jones has spent much time out in communal areas, enjoys watching "her programs" on TV in the early afternoon, has attended Baptist religious services in the chapel, group discussions, exercise class (only to watch, complains that the exercises are too painful), arts and craft classes (also, just to watch), and a few parties.  Mrs. Smith reports that Mrs. Jones used to crochet to pass time, and has brought in several items made by Mrs. Jones in years past, but resident has not been able to crochet for about two years — just about the same time her favorite granddaughter moved away to California.  Mrs. Smith and Mrs. Jones both talk about the beautiful gardens "I used to grow before I got crippled…"  Mrs. Jones seems friendly with many of the other residents, talks freely, initiates conversations, when in group discussion she will contribute her opinions and ideas about whatever the topic is for that day by prefacing each comment with phrases such as "I can't do that anymore, but…," "I really used to like that before I got put in this chair…," or "Those of us who are crippled should…."  Mrs. Smith stated on the third interview that her reasons for helping Mrs. Jones to move to a nursing facility was a hope that her mother could better accept herself in her current condition by being with other people her own age, with similar circumstances.  Mrs. Jones states the reason she has come to live in the home was because her daughter "no longer wanted to have a cripple around the house…I guess it was inevitable…"  When the two are together there seems to be an air of forced friendliness.  The daughter will greet her mother with a quick kiss on her cheek, ask how she is feeling, then start talking about one of her children before Mrs. Jones has a chance to respond to the question.  Usually any actual physical contact is limited to just the quick kiss on arrival and another at the end of the visit.  The two grandchildren who visit their grandmother use frequent touch, much hugging and hand holding.  Both mother and daughter state that it was Mrs. Jones' doctor's decision for her to enter the nursing facility.  Mrs. Jones helped decide which one by visiting several in the area before this admission.

**Problems And Needs:**
1.   Is exhibiting signs of low self-esteem, makes statements such as "Before I was crippled…" or "I used to be able to do…but I can't since I got stuck in this chair…"

2.  Uses pain as an excuse not to participate in exercise or in other activities which do not hold her interest.

3.  Needs to be evaluated further to determine appropriateness for some craft activities.

**Long Term Goal:**
Resident will adjust to life in the nursing facility.

**Short Term Goals:**
1.  Resident will increase self esteem as is evident by weekly participation in the volunteer beauty shop and participation in arthritis support group on Tuesday afternoons by the next update.

2.  Resident will agree to participate in yoga breathing classes for control of pain and for mild exercise by next update.

3.  Resident will agree to discuss participation in craft classes and allow evaluation by the next update.

**Approaches:**
1.  Activity Director will schedule resident for regular beauty shop appointments and will motivate resident to attend.

2.  Activity Director will include resident in yoga breathing classes for beginners.

3.  Reward active participation with much verbal praise. Encourage resident to use techniques learned in class when experiencing pain throughout the day.

4.  Activity Director will involve resident in arthritis discussion group. Motivate group to use peer pressure when resident makes self depreciating comments.  Inservice staff to reward positive statements about self with praise; ignore negative statements.

5.  Activity Director will evaluate resident for participation in craft classes.  One-on-one at first to determine if adaptive crochet

needle is appropriate.  Allow resident opportunities to discuss feelings regarding crochet interests.

6.   Activity Director or volunteer will involve resident in the following activities:

Baptist church services
Current events discussion group
Parties and scheduled entertainments
Good grooming classes and weekly manicures.

## Reassessment And Care Plan Update: (after the first 90 days)

(MDS quarterly review form continues to reassess Section N #1 and #2, "time awake" and "amount of time involved in activities."

| N. 1 | Time Awake | (Check appropriate time period over last 7 days.)<br><br>morning ☑        evening ☑<br>afternoon ☑        none ☐ |
|---|---|---|
| N. 2 | Average Time Involved in Activities | (When awake and not receiving tx. or ADL care )<br><br>0.  most - more than 2/3 of time        2.  little - less than 1/3 of time<br>1.  some - from 1/3 to 2/3 of time        3.  none        **1** |

Still this minimal reassessment does not reflect what is truly happening with Mrs. Jones.  Again, the importance of a narrative reassessment/progress note takes on even greater significance.)

Resident has shown some signs of increased self esteem, i.e., does not always preface her verbal participation in group discussion with negative statements about self and "crippled people."  These comments are usually only made when daughter, Mrs. Smith, is visiting. Tension continues during these visits, and nursing staff has noticed that most PRN pain medication is requested following these visits. Mrs. Jones does not express any verbal anger toward daughter, but it is obvious to staff that much anger is being experienced.  Arthritis support group has been somewhat helpful with confronting Mrs. Jones about her negative comments and letting her know that these are angry statements. So far Mrs. Jones has denied the anger, but seems to be more pensive the last few sessions when these discussions occur. Plan to continue with the support group and the reinforcement of staff when resident makes positive comments about self. Resident seems to really enjoy the special treatment she receives in the beauty shop, the manicure sessions, and the good grooming classes. Participation in yoga breathing classes is somewhat short of the participation resident agreed to in the last care plan. On discussing this with resident, Mrs. Jones verbalized a fear of having her doctor DC her PRN pain meds. Upon request the director of nursing talked with Mrs. Jones about this and reassured her that a decision like this would not be made without Mrs. Jones' input to the doctor. The DON encouraged Mrs. Jones to continue participation in the yoga classes. One-on-one's were scheduled to determine Mrs. Jones' physical ability to begin crocheting once again as a leisure pursuit. Mrs. Jones seemed unwilling at first to try the larger hook needles made available to her; she had "to discuss it" with her granddaughter in California. During the conversation with her granddaughter, resident learned she would become a great-grandmother near the end of the year. This news seemed to brighten her spirits and motivate her to try the crocheting once again. She is busy now working on a hand-crochet wall hanging for the baby's nursery using rug yarn and the large hook she refused at the beginning. When not busy in organized activities resident spends her time either working on the "baby rug" or visiting with others in the TV room. Grandchildren continue to visit at least two or three times a week. This is the highlight for Mrs. Jones. Resident is usually very verbal about her wants and desires and has expressed an interest in becoming more involved with a few of the residents who are "less fortunate than me..." See the changes in her care plan that follow.

**Problems And Needs:**
1.   Continues with much improvement. Continue goals and approaches.

2.   No longer uses pain as excuse not to participate, but still needs to be involved in yoga breathing classes and mild exercise.

3.   Needs to be kept supplied with rug yarn in "pretty pastel colors."

4.   Desires to become a resident volunteer.

**Short Term Goals:**
1.   Same

2.   Will continue to participate in yoga breathing classes on Monday, Wednesday, and Friday mornings until the next update. Will agree to try mild exercise class at least one time each week by the next update.

3.   Will continue to crochet daily, and will take responsibility for telling Activity Director when more yarns are needed until the next update.

4.   Will agree to visit three residents for the next two weeks and talk with Activity Director about which resident she will volunteer with on a three times a week basis. Will be responsible for her own volunteer time and will give a record of her volunteer visits to Activity Director before the next update of this care plan.

**Approaches:**
1.   Continues Approaches 1 - 4 from previous care plan.

2.   All staff to reward resident verbally with praise when Mrs. Jones makes positive statements about herself.

3.   Motivate resident to attend exercise classes on Tuesday mornings. Reward active participation with much praise.

4.   Activity Director will contact shopping volunteer and secure rug yarns as needed.

5.   Activity Director will assign three bedfast residents for Mrs. Jones to visit over the next two weeks. At the end of that time schedule a consultation to determine which of these residents Mrs. Jones will visit on a regular basis. Also, inservice Mrs.

Jones on how to keep a record of her time spent volunteering. Monitor the visits to determine suitability of this assignment.

6.   Continue with approach # 6 from previous plan.  Add Gardening Class.

## NOTE FROM THE AUTHOR:

As you can see by reading this case study, the care plan should read like a mini-history of the resident's life in the nursing facility.  Use the information in the next section of this book for a reference if you get stuck on what to write, or for ideas on how to cope with certain problems.  What is printed here is just a place to start.  Use it in that manner.  Do not be afraid to write, and do not budget your ink.  The best rule of thumb I have found over the last two decades has been: When in doubt, write it down; because if you don't, then it wasn't done…

For convenience in subdividing the section on sample care plan information, I have broken the information down according to the subheadings on the MDS.  You can use this information in one of the following ways:

1.   Review the information listed under each of the MDS subheadings.  Determine if the information is appropriate for your use; or,

2.   Look up the major diagnosis of the resident for whom you are writing your care plan and see if the information written under that subheading is of help; or,

3.   Use the Index in the back of this book.  Many of the problems and needs are listed alphabetically in the Index with the page numbers on which information about these problems and/or needs can be found.

I just can't stress enough the importance of involving your residents in the development of your, actually their, care plans as much as possible.  Only when you do this will you write a realistic care plan that will work — work both for you and for your residents.

# SECTION II

**Sample Problems/Needs,
Short Term Goals,
And Approaches**

# Delirium

Problems that may be triggered in this area indicate a sudden and/or recent change in the resident's behavior and/or response to his/her environment.

**Care Plan Information The Activity Director Could Use:**

**Problems/ Needs:** Sudden or recent onset of one or more of the following observed behaviors;

1. Less alert, easily distracted

2. Recent episodes of distorted thinking

3. Changing awareness of environment

4. Occasional/frequent incoherent speech

5. Rambling conversation

6. Periods of restless behavior, inability to sit still, hyperkinetic movements

7. Visual/auditory hallucinations

8. Falls asleep easily, lethargic

9. Noticeable mood swings

10. Cries easily, cries out suddenly, hollers, constantly making noise

11. Cognitive ability varies over the course of the day

12. Inability to focus attention

13. Forgetful, difficulty remembering

14. Changing ability to interact with others

**STG:** Resident will return to normal level cognitive functioning as is evidenced by _________________ (describe resident's normal behavior) by __________ (date).

**Approaches:**

1. Give information regarding R.O. i.e., day, time of day, current events, etc.

2. Use resident's name often, introduce self at each encounter.

3. Inservice staff on R.O. techniques

4. Discuss with family regarding recent loss of significant other.

5. Discuss with family, history of the observed behavioral changes.

6. Evaluate need for counseling.

7. Encourage continued routine of daily activities.

8. Encourage resident to relax participation in routine of daily activities until physical illness has been corrected.

9. Provide individual programming until resident is able to resume normal level of activity participation.

10. Provide small group activities that foster individual attention to resident's tolerance.

11. Evaluate for inclusion in memory group (activities designed to help participants increase ability to remember).

# Comatose

Cognitive Pattern - persistent vegetative state, not awake/aware of environment; no discernible level of consciousness.

Problems that may be triggered in this area include:

1.  skin breakdown; prone to pressure sore;

2.  dry mouth;

3.  needs total ADL care;

4.  osteoporosis, bones break easily;

5.  prone to contractures;

6.  weight loss, anorexia, at risk for malnutrition;

7.  unresponsive to most stimuli…

**Care Plan Information The Activity Director Could Use:**

**Problems/**   Unresponsive to most stimuli
**Needs:**

    **STG:**    Will respond to pleasant stimulation by ______________ (moving arms, fingers, legs, voluntarily opening eyes, moving head to source of stimulation, ______________ other) by ______________ (date).

**Approaches:**

1.  Encourage resident to move on own.

2.  Schedule individual visits for sensory stimulation.  Use soft, furry objects - rub resident's arm, forehead, back of hand with object.

3.    Talk with resident about experience of feeling object.

4.    Use pleasant smelling objects, pass under resident's nose, allowing time for fragrance of object to be inhaled by resident.

5.    Talk with resident about what he/she is smelling.

6.    Use pleasant tasting food item (soft/liquid on end of cotton swab).  Rub gently on resident's bottom lip.  Talk with resident about what he/she is tasting.

7.    Provide music/voice tapes. Talk with resident about what he/she is hearing.

8.    Read to resident (books, magazine articles, newspapers, etc.).

9.    Talk with resident regarding current events.  Allow time for resident to respond.  Speak as if resident were responding.

10.    Assume resident is able to hear and understand, use resident's name often, introduce self at each encounter.

11.    Explain each procedure before beginning, continually explain what is occurring as each procedure progresses.

12.    Open curtains — daytime; TV/radio on station __________ at __________ (time of day).

13.    Close curtains — nighttime; TV/radio off at __________ (time).

# Cognitive Loss/Dementia

Problems that may be triggered in this area include:

1.  not able to remember location of room, dining room, activity room, other areas of building;

2.  not able to remember names of others;

3.  not aware of current season of year, date: month, day, current year;

4.  not able to recognize own name;

5.  does not know, unable to remember names of staff, other residents, family, _________________ other;

6.  not able to remember information after five minutes; continually repeating questions;

7.  not able to remember/unaware he/she is in a nursing facility;

8.  forgets he/she has eaten, complains of being hungry;

9.  difficulty with long-term memory;

10.  difficulty with short-term memory;

11.  confused regarding time sequences;

12.  does not recognize lifelong friends, family;

13.  calls staff by family's names;

14.  not able to carry conversations; speech incoherent; "rabbit trails;"

15.  restless, unable to sit still, short attention span;

16.  cries easily, calls out, hollers;

17.  unable to make decisions when offered choices;

18.  does not seem able to dress self, groom self, feed self;

19.  unable to toilet self;

20.  makes inappropriate decisions regarding clothing, layers clothing, undresses self in public;

21.  does not remember how to use spoon, fork, knife, hairbrush, comb, toothbrush, etc.;

22.  may think he/she is someone else;

23.  may have paranoid thoughts;

24.  may have hallucinations;

25.  decreased interaction with others;

26.  easily frustrated;

27.  overly dependent on others;

28.  wanders;

29.  "scapegoated" by other residents;

30.  exhibits fear when touched or approached by others;

31.  at risk for weight loss…

**Care Plan Information The Activity Director Could Use:**

**Problems/ Needs:**  Not able to remember location of room, dining room, activity room, other areas of building.

**STG:**  Will be able to locate _______________ by _______________ (date).

**Problems/ Needs:** Not able to remember names of others.

**STG:** Will be able to identify___________ by ______________ (date).

**STG:** Will recognize _________________ (name) by giving direct eye contact by ___________ (date).

**Problems/ Needs:** Not aware of current season of year, date: month, day day, current year.

**STG:** Will be able to remember ___________________________ by ______________ (date)

**Problems/ Needs:** Not able to recognize own name.

**STG:** Will show recognition of own name by _______________ _________________________________________________ (describe behavior that will indicate resident recognizes own name) by ______________ (date).

**Problems/ Needs:** Does not know, unable to remember names of others; staff other residents, family, _________________ other.

**STG:** Will be able to remember name of__________________ (name, identify person) by ______________ (date).

**Problems/ Needs:** Not able to remember information after five minutes; continually repeating questions. Example "What time is it?..."

**STG:** Will be able to remember ___________________________ by ______________ (date).

**Problems/ Needs:** Not able to remember/unaware he/she is in a nursing facility.

**STG:** Will be able to make statement "I live in
_________________________ (name of facility) by
_______________ (date).

**Problems/
Needs:** Forgets he/she has eaten, complains of being hungry.

**STG:** Will be able to remember approximate time of last meal
by _______________ (date).

**Problems/
Needs:** Difficulty with long term memory.

**STG:** Will participate in reminiscence group _______________
(times weekly).

**Problems/
Needs:** Difficulty with short term memory.

**STG:** Will participate in memory group _______________
(times weekly).

**Problems/
Needs:** Resident confused regarding time sequences, i.e., "I
was born 1945, graduated high school 1930..."

**STG:** Resident will be able to remember _______________ by
_______________ (date).

**Problems/
Needs:** Does not recognize lifelong friends, family

**STG:** Resident will be able to recognize _______________ by
(date).

**Problems/
Needs:** Calls staff by family names.

**STG:** Will be able to remember name of ___________ by
_______________ (date).

**Problems/ Needs:** Not able to carry conversation; speech incoherent; "rabbit trails" (rambling conversation from one topic to another without apparent connection).

**STG:** Will be able to answer questions appropriately __________ number of times (3 of 5, 2 of 5, etc.) by _____________ (date).

**STG:** Will be able to speak about one topic for a ___________ (number of minutes) conversation by _____________ (date).

**STG:** Will be able to answer "yes" or "no" questions __________ number of times (3 of 5, 2 of 5, etc.) by _____________ (date).

**Problems/ Needs:** Restless, unable to sit still, short attention span; raps hands on table, in constant motion, wanders, fidgets with clothing.

**STG:** Will increase attention span to _____________ number of minutes by _______________ (date).

**STG:** Will be able to sit still for _____________ number of minutes by _______________ (date).

**STG:** Will rest _____________ number of minutes (every hour, every 2 hours, every 3 hours) by _____________ (date).

**STG:** Will remain dressed for ___________ number of hours per day by _______________ (date).

**STG:** Will limit changing of clothes to ___________ number of times per day by _______________ (date).

**STG:** Will be able to remain in _______________ (name of activity) for (___________ number of minutes, entire activity) by _____________ (date).

**Problems/ Needs:** Cries easily, calls out, hollers, constantly making verbal noises.

**STG:** Will be able to sit quietly for _______________ number of minutes by _______________ (date).

**Problems/ Needs:** Unable to make decisions when offered choices.

**STG:** Will be able to choose _______________ by _______________ (date).

**STG:** Will be able to accept decisions of others by _______________ (date).

**Problems/ Needs:** Makes inappropriate decisions regarding clothing i.e. wears shorts and T-shirt when 30° outside, etc. Layers clothing, undresses self in public.

**STG:** Will be appropriately dressed daily.

**STG:** Will be able to choose climate appropriate clothing by _______________ (date).

**STG:** Will choose one item of clothing to wear by _______________ (date).

**STG:** Will only wear _______________ numbers of layers of clothing at one time by _______________ (date).

**STG:** Will remain clothed when in public areas by _______________ (date).

**Problems/ Needs:** Does not remember how to use spoon, fork, knife, hairbrush, comb, toothbrush, _______________ other.

**STG:** Will be able to use _______________ by _______________ (date).

**STG:** Will be able to _______________ by _______________ (date).

**Problems/ Needs:** May think he/she is someone else.

**STG:** Will respond to own name ____________ number of times (2 of 5, 3 of 5, etc.) by ____________ (date).

**Problems/ Needs:** May have thoughts that others are "going to get me," "poison me"… etc.

**STG:** Will show sign of trusting others as evidenced by ____________ (describe behavior) by ____________ (date).

**Problems/ Needs:** May see and/or hear that which others do not see and/or hear.

**STG:** Will be aware of actual surroundings by ____________ (date).

**Problems/ Needs** Decreased interaction with others; impaired interaction with others.

**STG:** Will participate in conversation with ____________ (A.D., staff, volunteer, ____________ other) by ____________ (date).

**Problems/ Needs:** Difficulty making decisions; easily frustrated; overly dependent on others, etc.

**STG:** Will be able to make decision about sugar in coffee by ____________ (date).

**STG:** Will be able to make decision about ____________ by ____________ (date).

**STG:** Will remain calm during decision making by ____________ (date).

**STG:** Will be able to make decisions without cues from others by ____________ (date).

**Problems/**  Wanders around; needs constant supervision; often
**Needs:**  "scapegoated" by other residents; wanders into other
residents rooms; picks up items belonging to others.

**STG:**  Will have appropriate outlet for excess energy as is
evident by (only walking in approved areas, only walking in the hall, _____________ other) by _____________
(date).

**STG:**  Will only pick up items belonging to self by
_____________ (date).

**STG:**  Will spend "wandering time" in group setting with other
residents by _____________ (date).

**Problems/**  Exhibits fear when touched or approached by others.
**Needs:**

**STG:**  Will be able to trust (AD, nurse, nurse aide, volunteer,
_____________ other) as is evidenced by (not pulling
away from physical contact, not screaming when approached, not striking out at other person, _____________
other) by _____________ (date).

## Approaches:

1.   Use resident's name frequently during conversation, repeat phrases
as necessary.

2.   Gain resident's attention by speaking directly to him, maintain
eye contact, stand or sit close to resident, speak slowly and
clearly using concrete terms.

3.   Allow resident time to respond, be patient and firm.

4.   Reward appropriate responses with smiles, nod of head, and
verbal praise.

5.  One-on-one instruction on working with resident on (location of room, location of _______________________________, other; identification of ____________; remembering ____________).

6.  Ask "yes" and/or "no" type questions; allow time for resident to respond.

7.  Include resident in conversation; do not talk "about" him/her when he/she is present.

8.  Inservice staff to encourage resident to exercise choices in what clothing to wear — narrow choices to two or three items; allow resident to choose.

9.  Include resident in feeding group; encourage resident to eat with verbal phrases that are friendly and kind; do not hurry resident.

10. Set up meal service activity in intimate group of three to four residents in quiet area.

11. Serve each food item separately, in individual bowls — in courses one at a time.

12. Encourage self feeding, reminding and/or prompting resident as needed.

13. Do not scold resident during episodes of inappropriate behavior; offer gentle, but firm suggestions as to what is expected of resident.

14. Assign (volunteer, staff, family member, ____________ other) to stay with resident during group activities.

15. Assign (volunteer, ____________ other) to visit with resident to talk about events that occur in and around the nursing facility.

16. Be observant at all times of resident's movement, but do not restrain.

17.   Inservice staff to arrange personal items in same place in resident's room; encourage resident to use same.

18.   Explain any activity before beginning; use repetition as necessary; be warm and friendly.

19.   During episodes of hostility, allow resident to express self, but do not physically restrain unless resident attempts harm to self or others.

20.   Do not interfere when resident is arguing with another resident; be observant to any physical contact that may occur.

21.   Explain carefully to other residents to be more tolerant of this resident's behavior.

22.   Be supportive of family; educate family as to resident's constantly changing behavior, encourage continued contact with resident.

23.   Help resident to identify feelings by making statements such as "you sound angry," or "you sound upset"…

24.   Involve resident in the following activities:

   a.   One on one for sensory stimulation to work on ____________
   b.   Small group for sensory stimulation to work on __________
   c.   __________ Current events discussion
   d.   __________ Nature walks
   e.   __________ Sing-a-long
   f.   __________ Special exercise
   g.   __________ Special crafts
   h.   __________ Music listening
   i.   __________ Parties
   j.   __________ Entertainment
   k.   __________ Reminiscence group
   l.   __________ Validation therapy group
   m.   __________ Memory class

# Visual Function

Problems that may be triggered in this area include:

1.   needs large print books/magazines;

2.   unable to see to read;

3.   can only see with glasses;

4.   needs magnifying glass to read;

5.   only sees shadows; dark and light;

6.   needs glasses;

7.   totally blind;

8.   no depth perception; blind in one eye, difficulty ambulating;

9.   impaired vision, only sees objects to left (or to right);

10.  leaves food on plate because of vision problem;

11.  has artificial eye;

12.  unable to feed self because of lack of vision;

13.  feeds self with hands; spills food;

14.  doesn't recognize people;

15.  sees halos or rings around lights; sees flashes of light;

16.  offended by bright lights, glare;

17.  lost glasses; broke glasses;

18.  complains of pain in eyes;

19. unable to place glasses on face; unable to locate glasses;

20. redness, pain in eyes; complains of headaches;

21. complains of nausea, vomits;

22. complains of excessive dryness in eyes;

23. exhibits excessive tearing and/or mucous discharge in eyes;

24. needs assist getting to and from activity areas;

25. needs volunteers to read to resident;

26. needs talking book;

27. needs assistance during activities for full participation...

**Care Plan Information The Activity Director Could Use:**

**Problems/ Needs:**  Needs large print books/magazines.

**STG:**  Resident will be able to read.

**Problems/ Needs:**  Unable to see to read, enjoys literature.

**STG:**  Resident will be able to use talking books independently by _____________ (date).

**Problems/ Needs:**  Can only see with glasses.

**STG:**  Resident will wear glasses daily.

**Problems/ Needs:**  Needs magnifying glass to read.

**STG:**  Resident will be able to read.

**Problems/ Needs:** Only sees shadows; dark and light, enjoyed reading.

**STG:** Resident will be able to use talking books independently by ____________ (date).

**Problems/ Needs:** Needs to be evaluated for glasses.

**STG:** Evaluation will occur by ____________ (date).

**Problems/ Needs:** Totally blind

**STG:** Will maintain maximal independence as is evident by ____________ .

**STG:** Will be able to locate ____________ room by ____________ (date).

**STG:** Will be able to feed self by ____________ (date).

**STG:** Will be able to dress self by ____________ (date).

**STG:** Will be able to participate in ____________ activity (activities) by ____________ (date).

**Problems/ Needs:** Doesn't recognize people.

**STG:** Will be able to identify others using one or more of the other senses by ____________ (date).

**STG:** Will be able to recognize ____________________ by ____________ (date).

**Problems/ Needs:** Sees halos or rings around lights; sees flashes of light.

**STG:**  Will be able to maintain maximal independence as is evidenced by ______________ by ______________ (date).

**STG:**  Will be able to function within his/her environment with a minimum of discomfort as is evidenced by ______________ (behavior) by ______________ (date).

**STG:**  Will agree to physician's evaluation by ______________ (date).

**Problems/ Needs:**  Offended by bright lights, glare; unable to tolerate.

**STG:**  Will accept and wear dark glasses daily so as not to interfere with normal routine by ______________ (date).

**STG:**  Will wear sun visor daily.

**STG:**  Will wear dark glasses daily.

**Problems/ Needs:**  Lost glasses, broken glasses

**STG:**  Glasses will be (replaced, repaired) by ______________ (date).

**Problems/ Needs:**  Unable to place glasses on face; unable to locate glasses.

**STG:**  Resident will wear glasses daily.

**Problems/ Needs:**  Needs assistance getting to and from activity areas; has difficulty ambulating around nursing home.

**STG:**  Will attend ______________ (number) activities (with assist, without assist) weekly by ______________ (date).

**STG:**  Will be able to go from room to ______________ (area) by counting steps by ______________ (date).

**STG:**   Will use cane to ambulate around nursing facility by _______________ (date).

**Problems/**   Needs volunteer to read to resident.
**Needs:**

**STG:**   Will enjoy reading of volunteer by _______________ (date).

**Problems/**   Needs talking book machine and "books;" needs
**Needs:**   instruction on its use.

**STG:**   Will have talking books by _______________ (date).

**STG:**   Will be able to operate talking books per self by _______________ (date).

**Problems/**   Needs assistance during activities for full participation.
**Needs:**

**STG:**   Will participate in _______________ (activity, activities) with volunteer assistance by _______________ (date).

## Approaches:

1. Inservice staff to educate resident to his room and surrounding; help him to form a mental image of surroundings. Do not move items in room unnecessarily; educate/inform resident to any changes. Arrange clothing in color groups; educate resident. Encourage resident to maintain independence in (dressing, feeding, grooming, _______________ other). Identify food for resident using clock positions so he/she may feed self.

2. Orient resident to different areas of nursing facility; assist in counting of steps from area to area.

3. Make arrangements for transportation to see eye doctor.

4. Contact (family, _______________ other) regarding acquisition of eye glasses.

5. Secure large print books for resident's reading pleasure.

6. Treat resident as normal individual and allow freedom of movement.

7. When guiding resident, offer your arm for him/her to hold.

8. Assign volunteer to read to resident ______________ times (weekly, monthly).

9. Provide resident with magnifying glass, prism glasses, other.

10. Provide resident with large print reading material, bingo cards, playing cards, ______________ other.

11. Provide with talking book equipment; instruct on use.

12. Educate resident to any changes that may occur in location of furniture in nursing facility.

13. Involve resident in the following activities:

   a. ______________ Parties
   b. ______________ Religious services
   c. ______________ Discussion groups
   d. ______________ Sing-a-longs
   e. ______________ Current events
   f. ______________ Resident Council
   g. ______________ Pottery class (assist in choice of color for glazes
   h. ______________ Painting class (arrange colors on palette, identify location using clock positions)
   i. ______________ Entertainments
   j. ______________ Exercise and involvement
   k. ______________ Music listening
   l. ______________ Cards (secure large for visually impaired)
   m. ______________ Bingo (secure large print bingo cards)
   n. ______________ Cooking class (monitor for safety)
   o. ______________ Other

# Communication/Hearing

Problems that may be triggered in this area include:

1. able to only hear in quiet setting;

2. needs to be close to sound source to be able to hear;

3. unable to hear normal tones/sounds;

4. functionally deaf;

5. needs hearing evaluation;

6. wears hearing aid;

7. needs to read lips;

8. communicates through written messages;

9. wants to learn sign language; uses sign language;

10. aphasic;

11. needs communication board;

12. unable to speak English;

13. speech garbled and/or disjointed;

14. difficulty finishing thoughts, rambles;

15. communication limited to concrete messages;

16. has difficulty understanding others;

17. communicates with hand gestures;

18. complains of dizziness; vertigo;

19.  complains of ringing in ears;

20.  refuses opportunities to be with others;

21.  complains of pain in ears;

22.  refuses activities because of hearing loss;

23.  complains of "noises" which interfere with hearing;

24.  needs one-to-one communicator to talk with others;

25.  seems suspicious of others; withdrawn;

26.  insecure in unfamiliar surroundings;

27.  excessive wax in ear canal…

## Care Plan Information The Activity Director Could Use:

**Problems/**  Hearing impaired; able to only hear in quiet setting.
 **Needs:**

    **STG:**  Resident will be able to adequately hear by _____________
 (date).

    **STG:**  Will be evaluated for hearing aid usage by _____________
 (date).

**Problems/**  Needs to be placed close to sound source to be able to
 **Needs:**  hear.

    **STG:**  Resident will take responsibility for seating self close to
 sound source during activities _____________ (date)

    **STG:**  Resident will be able to adequately hear by _____________
 (date).

**Problems/**  Unable to hear normal tones/sounds.
 **Needs:**

**STG:**  Will be evaluated for hearing aid usage by ______________ (date).

**STG:**  Will be able to use hearing aid by ____________ (date).

**STG:**  Will be able to read lips by ____________ (date).

**Problems/ Needs:**  Unable to hear; functionally deaf.

**STG:**  Will be able to read lips by ____________ (date).

**STG:**  Will be able to communicate through use of sign language by ____________ (date).

**STG:**  Will be able to use hearing aid by ____________ (date).

**Problems/ Needs:**  Unable to hear; needs hearing evaluation.

**STG:**  Will be evaluated for hearing aid by ____________ (date).

**Problems/ Needs:**  Unable to hear; wears hearing aid in (right, left, both) ears.

**STG:**  Will be able to adequately hear daily.

**STG:**  Will be able to use hearing aid independently by ____________ (date).

**Problems/ Needs:**  Unable to hear; needs to be able to read lips.

**STG:**  Will be able to read lips by ____________ (date).

**STG:**  Will be able to read lips daily.

**Problems/ Needs:**  Unable to hear; is able to read written messages.

**STG:** Will be able to communicate with others by using written word by ______________ (date).

**Problems/ Needs** Resident wants to learn sign language; uses sign language to communicate.

**STG:** Resident will be able to communicate through use of sign language by ______________ (date).

**STG:** Will be able to communicate with staff by ______________ (date).

**Problems/ Needs:** Unable to comprehend verbal communications; has receptive aphasia.

**STG:** Will be able to use communication board by ______________ (date).

**STG:** Will be able to communicate basic needs by ______________ (date).

**Problems/ Needs:** Unable to communicate verbally; aphasic.

**STG:** Will be able to communicate basic needs through use of written word by ______________ (date).

**STG:** Will be able to communicate basic needs through use of "universal sign language."

**STG:** Will be able to communicate basic needs through use of communication board.

**Problems/ Needs:** Occasional conflicting communication — may say "yes" when means "no;" expressive aphasia.

**STG:** Will be able to communicate basic needs by ______________ (date).

**STG:** Will remember to use written word to communicate when conflicting messages interrupt communication.

**Problems/ Needs:** Communicates only using written messages.

**STG:** Will be able to communicate with staff daily.

**Problems/ Needs:** Needs communication board; unable to speak English; only speaks ____________ (language).

**STG:** Will be able to use communication board by ____________ (date).

**Problems/ Needs:** Difficulty making self understood; speech garbled and/ or disjointed.

**STG:** Will be able to communicate basic needs daily.

**STG:** Will be able to finish ____________ number sentences (2 of 5, 3 of 5, etc.) by ____________ (date).

**STG:** Will be able to communicate basic needs through use of communication board by ____________ (date).

**Problems/ Needs:** Difficulty finishing thoughts; rambles.

**STG:** Will be able to communicate basic needs by ____________ (describe behavior) by ____________ (date).

**Problems/ Needs:** Communication limited to simple, concrete messages.

**STG:** Will be able to communicate with others by ____________ (date).

**STG:** Will interact with ____________ number of people per day by ____________ (date).

**STG:**  Will continue to communicate with others daily.

**Problems/
Needs:**  Seems to have difficulty understanding others.

**STG:**  Will be able to understand others as is evidenced by ________________ (continued interaction with others, ____________ other) by ____________ (date).

**Problems/
Needs:**  Comprehension of others limited to gestures, universal language, pictures, ____________ other.

**STG:**  Will be able to communicate basic needs by ____________ (date).

**STG:**  Will be able to understand others as is evidenced by ____________ (continued interaction with others, ____________ other) by ____________ (date).

**Problems/
Needs:**  Refuses to participate in activities because of hearing loss.

**STG:**  Will participate in ____________ (number) of activities by ____________ (date).

**Problems/
Needs:**  Complains of "noises" which interfere with hearing.

**STG:**  Will understand conversations of others as is evidenced by talking with ____________ (number) others daily by ____________ (date).

**Problems/
Needs:**  Needs one-on-one communicator to talk with others.

**STG:**  Will talk with ____________ (number) of others with aid of one-on-one communicator by____________(date).

**Problems/
Needs:**  Seems suspicious of others; withdrawn because of hearing loss.

**STG:** Will interact with ______________ (number) others daily by ____________ (date).

**Problems/
Needs:** Insecurity at unfamiliar surroundings.

**STG:** Will feel comfortable in surroundings as is evidenced by ________________ (interaction with others, active participation in activity, ____________ other) by ____________ (date).

## Approaches:

1. Take time to communicate with resident.  Use short simple phrases; repeat as needed.  Allow time for resident to respond.

2. Place resident near source of sound, eliminate outside distractions as best possible.

3. Schedule resident for hearing evaluation with ____________ (name of resource for this service).

4. Place mouth close to resident's ear; lower tonal quality of voice; speakup, but do not shout.  Use short simple phrasing, repeat as needed.

5. Place hearing aid in ear; encourage resident to turn volume to level that enables him/her to hear.  Check batteries weekly or as needed; change prn.

6. Face resident when communicating; speak in normal tone - encourage resident to read lips.  Do not turn away from resident while speaking.

7. Communicate with resident by writing messages on paper with pencil/pen.  Provide resident with supply of paper and writing instruments.

8. Communicate with resident using gestures, drawing or using pictures.  Encourage resident to pay attention.

9.  Provide resident with communication board/cards portraying basic needs.  Teach resident to use.  Inservice staff on use of communication boards.

10.  Mirror resident's speech; i.e., repeat to resident what you have heard resident say.  Pay attention to gestures as well as phrases; attempts to understand.  Use Validation Therapy techniques.

11.  Provide speech therapy evaluation/provide therapy.

12.  Contact local resource for teaching sign language.  Enroll resident in these classes.

13.  Obtain sign language interpreter.

14.  Educate staff regarding basic sign language.

15.  Obtain interpreter for ____________ language.

16.  Encourage to interact with others, avoid isolation.

17.  Obtain telephone amplifier for resident's use; television closed-caption device; television amplifier; ____________ others.

18.  Position resident near sound source during activities. Encourage resident to take responsibility for this sort of placement.

19.  Use (one-on-one communicator, Port-a-Comm) when talking with resident; provide same for resident's use; instruction.

20.  Counsel with resident regarding feelings; encourage resident to verbalize feelings.

21.  Provide volunteer to visit in room with resident ____________ (number) times weekly.

22.  Instruct staff and other residents in importance of positioning self so resident may see facial expressions and read lips.

23. Never discuss resident with others in his/her immediate area.

24. Consult nursing to secure physician's order for hearing evaluation.

25. Arrange for audiologist to evaluate resident.

26. Include resident in the following activities:

    a. __________ Parties
    b. __________ Religious services
    c. __________ Cards and games
    d. __________ Cooking class
    e. __________ Friendly visitor
    f. __________ Crafts
    g. __________ Entertainments
    h. __________ Exercise and movement
    i. __________ Bingo
    j. __________ Resident volunteer program
    k. __________ Resident Council
    l. __________ Drawing class

# Physical Functioning and Structural Problems, Bed, Mobility, Transferring, Ambulation

Problems that may be triggered in this area include:

1.  unable to turn self in bed;

2.  unable to transfer self;

3.  unable to ambulate self;

4.  refuses to move self, turn self in bed;

5.  refuses to transfer self;

6.  unaware of body feelings, loss of tactile senses;

7.  cognitively unaware of need to move about;

8.  at risk for deterioration of mobility skills due to restraints...

**Care Plan Information The Activity Director Could Use:**

(Note: Problems and Goals will in all probability be set by nursing, physical therapy, and/or occupational therapy. The Activity Director may have input in the area of approaches.)

**Approaches:**

1.  Evaluate cognitive skills that may affect (mobility, transfer skills, ambulation ability).

2.  Remind resident to move (in bed, chair, _____________ other) every two hours or when at resident's bedside.

3.  Evaluate psychosocial needs that may affect desire to do for self.

4.  Teach resident proper use of wheelchair.

5.    Teach resident to use the clock as a means of remembering to move about, turn.

6.    Passive exercise to extremities at _______________ a.m. (time) and _______________ p.m.

7.    Include resident in daily bed exercise program.

# Dressing

Problems that may be triggered in this area include:

1. unable to dress self;

2. unable to make decisions regarding what to wear;

3. layers clothing, dresses inappropriate for temperature/climate;

4. undresses self in public; changes clothes often throughout the day;

5. needs assistance fastening clothing;

6. refuses to wear day clothes, shoes, etc.;

7. wears prosthesis, refuses to wear prosthesis.

**Care Plan Information The Activity Director Could Use:**

(Note: As in the other areas of ADL, the problems and goals will probably be set by nursing.  The Activity Director will have input primarily in the area of approaches.)

**Approaches:**

1. Monitor resident throughout day, redirect resident's attention when beginning to disrobe.  Encourage resident to remain clothed.

2. Monitor resident's dress in a.m., observe for climate appropriate dressing.  Gently cue resident as needed.  Reward appropriate dress with praise.

3. Monitor resident's dressing throughout the day.  Do not reward dress changes with compliments.  Encourage family to limit variety of available clothing each day.

4.   Teach resident in use of buttonhook to close buttons.

5.   Talk with family regarding substituting buttons/zippers with velcro closing.

6.   Talk with family regarding sturdy slip-on shoes or velcro-closed shoes.

7.   Include resident in activities that promote increased awareness of environment and environmental changes.

8.   Include resident in current events classes to increase awareness of environment.

# Eating

Problems that may be triggered in this area include:

1. unable to feed self;

2. refuses to feed self;

3. needs assistance with meals;

4. difficulty reaching the table, spills food;

5. feeds self with hands, not able/forgets how to use utensils;

6. unable to chew and swallow foods; difficulty swallowing;

7. plays with food; throws food;

8. eats from other resident's trays;

9. refuses to eat with other residents, prefers to eat alone.

**Care Plan Information The Activity Director Could Use:**

(Note: Problems and goals in this area may be set primarily by nursing and/or dietary.  The Activity Director's input would probably fall in the area of the approaches.)

**Approaches:**

1. Teach resident to use ___________________ (self-help device).

2. Visit with resident regarding dignity.

3. Include resident in feeding group activity to encourage independence in eating.

4. Provide resident with finger foods during activities, encourage resident to feed self.

5.  Visit with resident regarding eating alone versus eating in the dining room.  Seek reasons for refusal to eat in dining room.  Share information with appropriate parties.

# Toilet Use

Problems that may be triggered in this area include:

1.   unable to remain seated on toilet without supervision;

2.   does not remember to go to toilet;

3.   loss of sensation and/or urge to go toilet;

4.   unable to transfer self to toilet;

5.   unable to remove and then replace clothing for toilet use;

6.   unable to change and care for own use of sanitary napkins, incontinent pads, adult diaper, external catheter, etc.;

7.   unable to care for own colostomy, catheter, etc.,

8.   at risk for decline in toilet use due to arthritis, weakness, increasing dementia, ________________ other;

9.   unable to use toilet, bedpan, bedside commode, etc.

**Care Plan Information The Activity Director May Use:**

(Note: As in the other ADL areas, the problems and goals here will predominately be set by the nurse. The Activity Director might wish to add input in the area of the approaches.)

**Approaches:**

1.   Encourage resident to use the clock in remembering to go to bathroom, i.e. every two hours.

2.   Encourage resident to ask for assistance toileting as needed.

3.   Monitor resident for signs of discomfort that are indicative of an urge to use toilet such as ______________ (squirming in chair,

pulling on trousers, _________________ other).  Take to toilet as indicated.

4.    Request resident to be assisted to toilet before beginning activity.

5.    On outings with resident, remind and take to bathroom every ____________ (1-2 hours) or as needed.  Assist resident with clothing.

# Personal Hygiene and Bathing

Problems that may be triggered in this area include:

1.  unable to comb hair;

2.  unable to shave self;

3.  unable to brush teeth;

4.  unable to apply make-up;

5.  unable to wash hands, face, _____________ other, needs assistance;

6.  unable to bathe self...

**Care Plan Information The Activity Director May Use:**

(Note:  In this area, like the other areas of ADL, nursing is the predominate problem/goal setter.  The Activity Director's input falls mostly in the area of approaches.)

**Approaches:**

1.  Assist in evaluating physical abilities to determine reason for difficulty with _____________ (combing hair, shaving self, brushing teeth, applying make-up, washing hands, bathing, _____________ other).

2.  Evaluate cognitive abilities to determine ability to be self sufficient in ADL's.

3.  Provide brush and/or comb with a velcro strap.

4.  Provide universal cuff for use with _____________ (comb, brush, toothbrush, _____________ other).

5.  Teach resident independence in _____________ (combing hair, brushing teeth, applying make-up, washing hands, bathing, _____________ other).

6.  Schedule resident for beauty shop appointments __________ times each month.

7.  Include resident in manicure.

8.  Include resident in activities that foster good grooming such as:

    a.  __________ beauty shop
    b.  __________ manicures
    c.  __________ make-up classes
    d.  __________ hand-washing classes
    e.  __________ other

# Continence

Problems that may be triggered in this area include:

1.  incontinent of bladder;

2.  incontinent of bowels;

3.  has incontinent episodes _______ times per week;

4.  complains of frequent urination;

5.  has uncontrolled diarrhea;

6.  complains of pain on urinating;

7.  restrained daily, unable to toilet self;

8.  exhibits signs of urinary retention...

**Care Plan Information The Activity Director May Use:**

(Note:  The nurse will be identifying problems and goals in this area. The Activity Director may wish to add input in the area of approaches.)

**Approaches:**

1.  During activities offer resident opportunities to toilet self.

2.  Inform nurse of fluids consumed during activities (if resident uses catheter or is having record of input and output maintained.)

3.  Offer fluids during activities.

4.  Request resident be toileted before attending activities.

5.  Monitor catheter bag during activities, empty as needed.  Keep record of amount emptied, report to nursing.

# Psychosocial Well-Being

Problems that may be triggered in this area include:

1.   does not interact with others;

2.   does not initiate conversations with others;

3.   keeps others away by complaining;

4.   sits on fringe of group, doesn't talk with others;

5.   isolates self from others;

6.   refuses friendly advances of others;

7.   fidgets, moves away from others;

8.   does not wish to be included in group activities;

9.   uses somatic complaints as excuse not to participate in activities;

10.  does not pursue leisure activities during free time;

11.  complains of inability to talk with others;

12.  ill at ease with all residents;

13.  not able to make friends;

14.  thinks other residents are "crazy;"

15.  refuses to discuss former hobbies, leisure pursuits; states "I can't do that now…;"

16.  complains, "Staff does not understand me…;"

17.  disrupts group situation, yells at others, argues with others;

18.  argues with staff regarding daily routine;

19.  makes derogatory comments regarding other residents, staff;

20.  complains about roommate;

21.  expresses anger regarding nursing facility placement;

22.  argues with family members;

23.  does not exhibit understanding of others feelings;

24.  makes statements like "I'm so alone…" or "I feel left behind…;"

25.  has no family to visit;

26.  has outlived immediate family;

27.  has recently lost significant other;

28.  enjoys talking about past accomplishments;

29.  seems upset when talking about the past;

30.  isolates self because of hearing impairment, communication difference, ________________ other;

31.  does not interact with others because of age difference…

**Care Plan Information The Activity Director May Use:**

**Problems/ Needs:** Resident does not interact with others (staff, residents, family, volunteers, ____________ other).

**STG:** Resident will agree to talk with (activity director, ____________ other) ____________ times per (day, week, month) by ____________ (date).

**STG:** Resident will talk with (roommate, other residents, volunteers, ____________ other) ____________ times per day by ____________ (date).

**STG:** Resident will attend ________________ (name activity) ______________ times by ____________ (date).

**Problems/ Needs:** Resident does not initiate conversation with others.

**STG:** Resident will talk with ____________ number others ______________ times day by ____________ (date).

**STG:** Resident will answer questions of others (1 of 5, 2 of 5, ______________ other) times daily by ____________ (date).

**STG:** Resident will initiate conversation with (Activity Director, ____________ other) by ____________ (date).

**STG:** Resident will initiate conversation with others by ______________ (date).

**Problems/ Needs:** Resident keeps others away by complaining about ______________ (describe behavior).

**STG:** Resident will agree to talk with Activity Director regarding behavior by ____________ (date).

**STG:** Resident will decrease complaints to ______________ times per day by ____________ (date).

**STG:** Resident will complain when experiencing disappointment/deception only by ____________ (date).

**STG:** Resident will show enjoyment when talking with others as evidenced by ____________ (describe behavior).

**Problems/ Needs:** Resident sits on fringe of group, doesn't talk with others.

**STG:** Resident will place self next to other resident during group situation by ____________ (date).

**STG:** Resident will show participation in group activity by ______________ (nodding head, responding to questions of others, talking, ______________ other) by ______________ (date).

**Problems/ Needs:** Resident spends many hours sitting away from others in ______________ (name, place).

**STG:** Resident will agree to (talk, communicate) with activity director, volunteer, staff, other resident, ______________ other) ______________ times day by ______________ (date).

**STG:** Resident will agree to sit close to other resident for ______________ number minutes per day by ______________ (date).

**Problems/ Needs:** Resident avoids talking with others by ______________ (describe behavior).

**STG:** Resident will share reasons for avoidance with (activity director, ______________ other) by ______________ (date).

**STG:** Resident will accept friendly advances of other residents by ______________ (date).

**STG:** Resident will talk with ______________ number of others by ______________ (date).

**Problems/ Needs:** Resident refuses friendly advances of others by ______ ______________ (describe behavior).

**STG:** Resident will share reasons for refusal with (activity director ______________ other) by ______________ (date).

**STG:** Resident will talk with other residents by ______________ (date).

**Problems/ Needs:** Resident fidgets, moves away from others when in group situation.

**STG:**  Resident will keep place in group when other residents move next to resident by ____________ (date).

**STG:**  Resident will stay in group activity for ____________ % of activity by ____________ (date).

**Problems/ Needs:**  Resident does not wish to be included in group activities.

**STG**:  Resident will agree to discuss with (activity director, ____________ other) reasons for refusal by ____________ (date).

**STG:**  Resident's wishes will be respected, resident will agree to one-on-one activity with (activity director, ____________ other) by ____________ (date).

**STG:**  Resident will agree to try ____________ (name activity of interest) ____________ times per (month, week) by ____________ (date).

**Problems/ Needs:**  Resident uses somatic complaints as excuse not to participate in activities.

**STG:**  Resident will agree to discuss activity interests with activity director by ____________ (date).

**STG:**  Resident will agree to try ____________ (name activity of interest) ____________ times per (month, week) by ____________ (date).

**Problems/ Needs:**  Resident attends group activities, does not pursue leisure activities during free time.

**STG:**  Resident will agree to discuss leisure interests with activity director by ____________ (date).

**STG:**  Resident will agree to ____________ (read a magazine, watch TV, talk with friends on phone, ____________ other) one time a day by ____________ (date).

**Problems/ Needs:**  Resident complains of inability to communicate with other residents.

**STG:**  Resident will agree to discuss feelings with (activity director, ______________ other) by ______________ (date).

**STG:**  Resident will make one friend by ______________ (date).

**Problems/ Needs:**  Resident seems ill at ease with other residents, ________ ______________ (describe observed behavior).

**STG:**  Resident will agree to discuss feelings with (activity director, ______________ other) by ______________ (date).

**STG:**  Resident will talk with one other resident with similar interest by ______________ (date).

**STG:**  Resident will make one friend by ______________ (date).

**Problems/ Needs:**  Resident has not been able to make friends with other residents.

**STG:**  Resident will agree to talk with (activity director ______________ other) by ______________ (date).

**STG:**  Resident will agree to talk with ______________ (another resident with similar interests, volunteer, ______________ other) by ______________ (date).

**STG:**  Resident will make one friend by ______________ (date).

**Problems/ Needs:**  Resident states other residents are "crazy;" refuses opportunities to associate.

**STG:**  Resident will agree to talk with (activity director, ______________ other) regarding feelings by ______________ (date).

**STG:** Resident will show tolerance of other residents by talking with ____________ number of other residents per day by ____________ (date).

**STG:** Resident will find one other resident to call "friend" by ____________ (date).

**Problems/ Needs:** Resident refuses to discuss former hobbies, leisure pursuits; states "I can't do that now…"

**STG:** Resident will agree to discuss feelings with (activity director, ____________ other) by ____________ (date).

**STG:** Resident will share former hobbies, leisure pursuits information with activity director by ____________ (date).

**STG:** Resident will agree to try ____________ (name adaptive activity) by ____________ (date).

**STG:** Resident will ____________ (name activity) ____________ times per (week, day) by ____________ (date).

**Problems/ Needs:** Resident complains, "Staff does not understand me…"

**STG:** Resident will agree to discuss feelings with (activity director, ____________ other) by ____________ (date).

**STG:** Resident will be able to state, "Staff does try to understand me…" by ____________ (date).

**Problems/ Needs:** Resident disrupts group situations by ____________ (yelling at others, arguing with others, ____________ other).

**STG:** Resident will agree to sit quietly in group situation for ____________ number of minutes by ____________ (date).

**STG:**  Resident will increase tolerance of group situations and be able to sit for _____________ (number) minutes without disruptions by _____________ (date).

**STG:**  Resident will ask to leave group situation when desires by _____________ (date).

**Problems/Needs:**  Resident argues with staff regarding daily routine especially at_____________ (bathtime, mealtime,_____________ other).

**STG:**  Resident will agree to discuss feelings with (activity director _____________ other) by _____________ (date).

**STG:**  Resident will discuss preferences regarding_____________ (bathtime, meals,_____________ other) by _____________ (date)

**STG:**  Resident will agree to _______________ (bathe, eat, _____________ other) by _____________ (date) without arguing with staff.

**Problems/Needs:**  Resident makes derogatory comments regarding other residents, staff.

**STG:**  Resident will agree to discuss feelings behind comments with activity director _____________ (other) by _____________ (date).

**STG:**  Resident will agree to keep opinions private by _____________ (date).

**STG:**  Resident's tolerance of others will increase as evidenced by no derogatory or offensive comments made by _____________ (date).

**Problems/Needs:**  Resident complains about roommate, states_____________ (describe complaints/summarize complaints).

**STG:** Resident will discuss feelings with (activity director ___________ other) by ___________ (date).

**STG:** Resident will be able to state "I can accept my roommate…" by ___________ (date).

**STG:** Resident will be able to "make friend" with new roommate by ___________ (date).

**STG:** Resident will be able to verbalize one positive statement regarding roommate by ___________ (date).

**Problems/ Needs:** Resident expresses anger regarding nursing facility placement.

**STG:** Resident will agree to discuss feelings with (activity director, ___________ other) by ___________ (date).

**STG:** Resident will be able to state "I'm angry with ___________(daughter, son, ___________ other) for putting me here…" by ___________ (date).

**STG:** Resident will be able to express anger through participation in ___________ (name activity that facilitates appropriate release of angry feelings) by ___________ (date).

**STG:** Resident will be able to make one positive statement regarding nursing facility placement by ___________ (date).

**Problems/ Needs:** Resident has been observed arguing with family members when they visit.

**STG:** Resident will agree to discuss feelings with (activity director ___________ other) by ___________ (date).

**STG:** Resident will be able to express anger through participation in _____________ (name activity that facilitates appropriate release of angry feelings) by _____________ (date).

**STG:** Resident will be able to state "I was angry with _____________ (daughter, son, _____________ other) but now I've let the anger go…" by _____________ (date).

**Problems/ Needs:** Resident does not exhibit understanding of others feelings.

**STG:** Resident will agree to discuss feelings with (activity director, _____________ other) by _____________ (date).

**STG:** Resident will agree to think before speaking by _____________ (date).

**STG:** Resident will be able to state "Other residents have feelings, too…" by _____________ (date).

**Problems/ Needs:** Resident makes statements like "I'm so alone…" or "I feel left behind…"

**STG:** Resident will agree to discuss feelings with (activity director _____________ other) by _____________ (date).

**STG:** Resident will be able to state "I can still make friends…" by _____________ (date).

**STG:** Resident will be able to make friends with _____________ (number) other resident(s) by _____________ (date).

**Problems/ Needs:** Resident makes statements like "My daughter/son doesn't want to be bothered with me…" or "After all I've done for _____________ (name relation) she's/he's put me here…"

**STG:** Resident will agree to discuss feelings with (activity director, ______________ other) by ______________ (date).

**STG:** Resident will be able to express feelings to ______________ (son, daughter, ______________ other) by ______________ (date).

**STG:** Resident will be able to state, "I understand I may not like it, but I do understand ______________ " by ______________ (date).

**Problems/ Needs:** Resident has no family to visit/family only able to visit ______________ times (month, year) because of distance.

**STG:** Resident will have "adopted family" by ______________ (date).

**STG:** Resident will be able to state, "I may have no close family, but I do have friends..." by ______________ (date).

**STG:** Resident will talk with family ______________ times (month, week) via telephone by ______________ (date).

**STG:** Resident will communicate with family by mail ______________ times (month, week) by ______________ (date).

**Problems/ Needs:** Resident has outlived immediate family.

**STG:** Resident will have "adopted family" by ______________ (date).

**STG:** Resident will be able to state, "I may have no close family, but I do have friends..." by ______________ (date).

**STG:** Resident will make one new friend by ______________ (date).

**Problems/
Needs:**  Resident has recently experienced loss of _____________ (wife, husband, daughter, son, significant other, room-mate, _____________ other).

**STG:**  Resident will proceed through the grief process and discuss feelings as needed.

**STG:**  Resident will agree to discuss loss with (activity director, _____________ other) by _____________ (date).

**Problems/
Needs:**  Resident enjoys talking about past accomplishments particularly _____________ (summarize topic).

**STG:**  Resident will talk about _____________ (topic) _____________ times (week, day) by _____________ (date).

**STG:**  Resident will participate in discussion group/reminiscence group _____________ times (week, month) by _____________ (date).

**STG:**  Resident will make friends with _____________ (number) others with similar interests by _____________ (date).

**Problems/
Needs:**  Resident seems upset when talking about the past and past accomplishments _____________ (cries, sobs, _____________ other).

**STG:**  Resident will agree to discuss feelings with (activity director _____________ other) by _____________ (date).

**STG:**  Resident will be able to talk about the past without _____________ (crying, sobbing, _____________ other) by _____________ (date).

**Problems/
Needs:**  Resident makes statements like, "I'm not the person I used to be...," "I wish I had been a better _____________ (teacher, mother, father, _____________ other)...," or "I can't do that anymore..."

**STG:**  Resident will agree to discuss feelings with (activity director, _____________ other) by _____________ (date).

**STG:**  Resident will take an interest in self and will go to beauty shop _____________ times a month by _____________ (date).

**STG:**  Resident will agree to try _____________ (name activity) using adaptive (rules, devices, _____________ other) by _____________ (date).

**STG:**  Resident will be able to state, "I did the best I knew how..." by _____________ (date).

**Problems/ Needs:**  Resident sits away from others because of _____________ (communication difference, hearing impairment, _____________ other).

**STG:**  Resident will be able to sit next to one person for _____________ (length of time) by _____________ (date).

**STG:**  Resident will be able to communicate with one other person by _____________ (date).

**STG:**  Resident will be able to make friends with one other resident and establish means of communicating by _____________ (date).

**Problems/ Needs:**  Resident does not interact with others because of age difference.

**STG:**  Resident will agree to discuss feelings regarding age difference with (activity director, _____________ other) by _____________ (date).

**STG:**  Resident will make friends with volunteer of similar age by _____________ (date).

**STG:**  Resident will invite friends from outside the nursing facility to visit _____________ times (week, month) by _____________ (date).

## Approaches:

1. Visit with resident in private area.  Allow time for resident to express feelings.

2. Provide therapeutic counseling.

3. Offer resident opportunities to talk regarding thoughts and feelings.  Listen attentively.

4. Introduce resident to other residents.

5. Use names of others while speaking to assist resident in remembering names.

6. Visit with resident, talk about resident's interest in _____________ (name interest).

7. Be friendly, initiate conversation with friendly opening: "Hi, my name is _____________ ; How are you doing today…"

8. Invite resident to _____________ (name activity), encourage resident to "just listen."  After attending a few sessions, attempt to include resident in conversation — ask closed questions at first, work into open questions such as, "What do you think about…" or "Tell me about…"

9. Schedule resident for beauty shop appointments, encourage resident to attend.

10. Encourage roommate to assist in motivating resident to attend activities.

11. Introduce resident to other residents with similar interest. Enlist these other residents to assist in motivating resident to attend activities.

12. Talk with resident about the problems associated with dementia. Encourage resident to be patient.

13. Confront inappropriate behavior as such. Encourage resident to be assertive regarding needs and feelings. Discourage aggressive behavior.

14. Ignore aggressive behavior. Use much verbal praise when appropriate behavior is exhibited.

15. Explore possible reasons behind argumentative behavior. Eliminate causes.

16. Explore causes for problems with roommate, attempt to mediate discussion between resident and roommate.

17. HCP evaluate offering resident opportunity to change room. Enlist resident assistance in finding new roommate.

18. Involve resident in "New Resident's Support Group."

19. Involve resident in _____________ support group.

20. Recruit adopted family to visit with resident.

21. Involve resident in Adopt a Grandchild program.

22. Include resident in intergenerational programs.

23. Schedule one-on-one visits, monitor grief process. Encourage resident to express feelings.

24. Initiate contact with faraway family members via ___________ (mail, telephone).

25. Assist resident in responding to mail by offering to write letters dictated by resident.

26. Arrange for once a month/week phone calls with family.

27.  Involve resident in ______________ discussion group.

28.  Motivate group to exert peer pressure when resident makes self-depreciating comments.

29.  Inservice staff to reward positive statements about self with praise; ignore negative statements.

30.  Provide resident with ______________ (communication board, one-on-one communicator, ______________ other) to increase communication with others.

31.  Refer resident to audiologist for hearing evaluation.

32.  Recruit volunteers in resident's age range, introduce to resident. Encourage visits.

33.  Encourage resident to invite friends from home to visit nursing facility.

34.  Plan outings to include resident and offer opportunities to interact with the community.

35.  Include resident in the following act:

| | | |
|---|---|---|
| a. | __________ | Exercise class |
| b. | __________ | Reminiscence group |
| c. | __________ | Remotivation group |
| d. | __________ | Current events discussion |
| e. | __________ | Music listening |
| f. | __________ | Music classes |
| g. | __________ | Cooking class |
| h. | __________ | Crafts |
| i. | __________ | Bible study |
| j. | __________ | Support group |
| k. | __________ | Religious services |
| l. | __________ | Lecture series |
| m. | __________ | Yoga breathing class |
| n. | __________ | Sing-a-long |

o. __________ Outside trips
p. __________ Bingo
q. __________ Dominoes
r. __________ Checkers
s. __________ Darts
t. __________ Horseshoes
u. __________ Resident Council
v. __________ Other

36. Reward attendance/participation with verbal praise, warm smile.

# Mood and Behavior

Problems that may be triggered in this area include:

1.  sighs often;

2.  cries;

3.  looks dejected, unhappy when alone;

4.  expresses fear;

5.  jumps when touched;

6.  cries out, pulls away from staff;

7.  has flat affect, exhibits no changes in facial expression;

8.  states, "I feel worthless…" or "I feel like a nothing…;"

9.  states, "I feel guilty…;"

10. stays to himself/herself, isolates self in room;

11. becomes short of breath when upset;

12. paces in halls, outside;

13. appears to be in constant motion;

14. refuses to eat, refuses fluids;

15. refuses medications;

16. has stopped combing hair, wearing makeup/shaving;

17. refuses to wear day clothes;

18. expresses much anxiety regarding current health status;

19.  expresses desire to die;

20.  in sad mood, does not respond to attempts of others to "cheer-up;"

21.  makes angry statements;

22.  curses and yells at others;

23.  attempts to hit, scratch, spit on staff, other residents;

24.  has made sexual advances toward another resident;

25.  screams for no apparent reason;

26.  masturbates in public;

27.  grabs staff, other residents in sexually inappropriate manner;

28.  disrobes in public;

29.  goes in and out of other resident's rooms without invitation;

30.  rummages through the belongings of others;

31.  takes belongings of others without permission;

32.  hoards food in room;

33.  hoards paper trash;

34.  resists staff during care giving activities;

35.  refuses to change clothes;

36.  seems quiet, has had recent roommate change…

**Care Plan Information The Activity Director May Use:**

**Problems/**   Resident observed to sigh often; cries; looks dejected
  **Needs:**   unhappy when alone.

**STG:** Resident will agree to discuss feelings with (activity director _____________ other) by _____________ (date).

**Problems/ Needs:** Resident expresses fear; jumps when touched; cries out, pulls away from staff.

**STG:** Resident will agree to discuss feelings with (activity director _____________ other) by _____________ (date).

**STG:** Resident will remain calm when touched/approached by other residents or staff by _____________ (date).

**STG:** Resident will begin to trust staff as is evident by absence of _____________ (jumping when touched, crying out, pulling away, _____________ other) by _____________ (date).

**Problems/ Needs:** Resident has flat affect; exhibits no changes in expression due to _____________ (explain possible reasons).

**STG:** Resident will be able to verbally express feelings in absence of facial ability to show feelings by _____________ (date).

**STG:** Resident will be able to smile when feeling good; frown when feeling sad by _____________ (date).

**STG:** Resident will agree to discuss thoughts and feelings with (activity director, _____________ other) by _____________ (date).

**Problems/ Needs:** Resident states, "I feel worthless..." or "I feel like a nothing..."

**STG:** Resident will agree to discuss feelings with (activity director, _____________ other) by _____________ (date).

**STG:** Resident will not harm self or others over the next 90 days.

**STG:**  Resident will be able to state "I'm okay..."

**Problems/**
**Needs:**  Resident states "I feel guilty..."

**STG:**  Resident will agree to discuss feelings with (activity director ____________ other) by ____________ (date).

**STG:**  Resident will be able to identify actions which cause guilty feelings by ____________ (date).

**STG:**  Resident will be able to state "I'm okay..."

**Problems/**
**Needs:**  Resident stays to himself/herself; isolates self in room.

**STG:**  Resident will agree to talk with (activity director, ____________ other) by ____________ (date).

**STG:**  Resident will agree to accept ____________ (number) of visits from other residents each week by ____________ (date).

**STG:**  Resident will agree to spend ____________ (number of minutes/hours) out of his/her room ____________ times (day, week) by ____________ (date).

**STG:**  Resident will agree to come to ____________ activity ____________ times (day, week, month) by ____________ (date).

**Problems/**
**Needs:**  Resident becomes short of breath when upset; has experienced SOB episodes ____________ times per week in last 30 days.

**STG:**  Resident will take responsibility for self and will remember to breathe deeply when upset by ____________ (date).

**STG:**    Episodes of SOB will decrease to ___________ times per week by ___________ (date).

**STG:**    Resident will be able to express feelings verbally when upset by ___________ (date).

**Problems/Needs:**    Resident paces in hallways, outside.

**STG:**    Resident will remember to rest when needed over next 90 days.

**STG:**    Resident will express feelings verbally by ___________ (date).

**STG:**    Resident will recognize pacing signifies that he/she is (upset/angry/ ___________ other) and verbalize feelings by ___________ (date).

**STG:**    Resident will agree to discuss feelings with (activity director, ___________ other) by ___________ (date).

**Problems/Needs:**    Resident appears to be in constant motion.

**STG:**    Resident will rest ___________ times per day for ___________ minutes by ___________ (date).

**STG:**    Resident will agree to talk with (activity director, ___________ other) by ___________ (date).

**Problems/Needs:**    Resident wanders around nursing home with no particular direction. When asked expresses, "I'm just (upset/bored/ ___________ other)…"

**STG:**    Resident will recognize wandering behavior signifies he/she is ___________ (upset, angry, bored, ___________ other) by ___________ (date).

**STG:** Resident will express feelings verbally by ______________ (date).

**STG:** Resident will agree to discuss feelings with (activity director, ______________ other) by ______________ (date).

**STG:** Resident will rest ______________ times per day for ______________ minutes by ______________ (date).

**STG:** Resident will agree to attend ______________ activities ______________ times (day, week) by ______________ (date).

**Problems/ Needs:** Resident refuses to eat, refuses fluids.

**STG:** Resident will agree to discuss reasons for refusal with (activity director, ______________ other) by ______________ (date).

**Problems/ Needs:** Resident refuses to take medications.

**STG:** Resident will be knowledgeable of consequences of refusal to take medications and make appropriate decision for self by ______________ (date).

**STG:** Resident will agree to continue life sustaining medication over next 90 days.

**STG:** Resident agrees to discuss reasons for refusal with (activity director, ______________ other) by ______________ (date).

**STG:** Resident will agree to take medications daily as ordered by physician over next 90 days.

**Problems/ Needs:** Resident has recently stopped combing hair, wearing makeup, shaving, ______________ other.

**STG:** Resident will agree to discuss reasons for change in ADL pattern with (activity director, ____________ other) by ____________ (date).

**STG:** Resident will agree to discuss feelings with (activity director, ____________ other) by ____________ (date).

**Problems/ Needs:** Resident refuses to wear day clothes.

**STG:** Resident will make own decisions regarding dress each day over next 90 days.

**STG:** Resident will agree to wear day clothes ____________ days per week by ____________ (date).

**Problems/ Needs:** Resident expresses much anxiety regarding current health status; makes statements like, "I'm not getting better…;" "I feel sick…," etc.

**STG:** Resident will agree to discuss fears with (activity director, ____________ other) by ____________ (date).

**STG:** Resident will be able to state, "I'm okay…" by ____________ (date).

**Problems/ Needs:** Resident makes statements like, "I'm having a heart attack…," "The cancer is coming back…," "I'm dying…," etc.

**STG:** Resident will agree to discuss feelings/fears with (activity director, ____________ other) by ____________ (date).

**STG:** Resident will be able to state, "I'm okay…" by ____________ (date).

**Problems/ Needs:** Resident expresses desire to die, makes statements like, "I wish I was dead…," "If I could just get my hands on a gun…," "No one should have to live like this…," etc.

**STG:** Resident will agree to discuss feelings with (activity director ______________ other) by ______________ (date).

**STG:** Resident will be able to state, "I'm okay…," by ______________ (date).

**Problems/ Needs:** Resident does not "cheer-up," does not respond to attempts of others to "cheer-up" overall sad mood for past ______________ days.

**STG:** Resident will agree to discuss feelings with (activity director, ______________ other) by ______________ (date).

**Problems/ Needs:** Resident makes angry statements to ______________ (staff, other resident, ______________ other).

**STG:** Resident will agree to discuss feelings with (activity director, ______________ other) by ______________ (date).

**STG:** Resident will attend ______________ activity to release physical energy of anger ______________ times week by ______________ (date).

**STG:** Resident will agree to take responsibility for feelings and discuss same in assertive manner by ______________ (date).

**STG:** Resident will direct anger into appropriate outlet such as ______________ (name activity) ______________ times week by ______________ (date).

**Problems/ Needs:** Resident curses and yells at others.

**STG:** Resident will agree to discuss feelings with (activity director, ____________ other) by ____________ (date).

**STG:** Resident will understand others do not enjoy being cursed or "yelled at" and will decrease to less than ____________ number episodes per (week, day) by ____________ (date).

**STG:** Resident will direct anger into appropriate outlet such as ____________ (name activity) ____________ times week by ____________ (date).

**Problems/ Needs:** Resident has been observed trying to hit other residents, attempts to ____________ (hit, scratch, spit on, ____________ other) staff.

**STG:** Resident will take responsibility for feelings and verbalize (anger, fear, ____________ other) by ____________ (date).

**STG:** Resident will attend ____________ (name activity) to release physical energy of anger ____________ times week by ____________ (date).

**STG:** Resident will agree to talk with (activity director, ____________ other) ____________ times week over the next 90 days.

**Problems/ Needs:** Resident has made sexual advances toward another ____________ (male, female) resident.

**STG:** Resident will keep activity to private area over next 90 days.

**STG:** Decision of two consenting adults will be respected over next 90 days.

**STG:** Resident will respect the right of the ____________ (male, female) resident to say "No" over next 90 days.

**STG:** Resident will agree to approach only those residents who are able to respond with consent over the next 90 days.

**Problems/ Needs:** Resident screams out for no apparent reason.

**STG:** Resident will decrease screams to ____________ times per (day, week) by ____________ (date).

**STG:** Resident will verbalize feelings behind screams by ____________ by ____________ (date).

**STG:** Resident will express feelings behind screams by ____________ (name activity) by ____________ (date).

**Problems/ Needs:** Resident masturbates in public.

**STG:** Resident will maintain privacy during masturbation prn.

**STG:** Resident will seek assistance from staff in obtaining privacy for activities over the next 90 days.

**STG:** Resident's dignity will be observed daily.

**Problems/ Needs:** Resident grabs ____________ (staff, other residents) in sexual advances in an inappropriate manner.

**STG:** Resident will understand others do not wish to be touched by ____________ (date).

**STG:** Resident's behavior will decrease to less than ____________ number of episodes per ____________ (week, day) by ____________ (date).

**STG:** Resident will find appropriate partner for his/her attention by ____________ (date).

**Problems/ Needs:**   Resident disrobes in public areas.

**STG:**   Resident will only change clothing in privacy of his/her room by ____________ (date).

**STG:**   Resident will be aware of surroundings and seek privacy to change clothing by ____________ (date).

**Problems/ Needs:**   Resident goes in and out of other resident's rooms without invitation.

**STG:**   Resident will respect privacy of others and not go into room with closed doors over the next 90 days.

**STG:**   Resident will agree to wait for invitation to enter other resident rooms over next 90 days.

**Problems/ Needs:**   Resident rummages through the belongings of others.

**STG:**   Resident will respect privacy of others and not rummage through their belongings over next 90 days.

**STG:**   Resident will attend ____________ (name activity providing appropriate outlet for need to rummage) ____________ times week by ____________ (date).

**Problems/ Needs:**   Resident takes belongings of others without permission.

**STG:**   Resident will respect rights of other residents and not take their belongings over next 90 days.

**STG:**   Resident will attend ____________ (name activity) ____________ times week by ____________ (date).

**Problems/ Needs:**   Resident hoards food in room; hoards paper trash.

**STG:**  Resident will be able to talk about ____________ (food, trash) by ____________ (date).

**STG:**  Resident will express reasons for keeping ____________ (food, trash) by ____________ (date).

**STG:**  Resident will be able to control hoarding by decreasing episodes to ____________ times per (week, month) by ____________ (date).

**Problems/ Needs:**  Resident resists staff during care giving activities.

**STG:**  Resident will allow staff to perform care giving activities daily over the next 90 days.

**STG:**  Resident will establish trust in staff providing care by decreasing resistance to ____________ number of episodes per ____________ (day, week) by ____________ (date).

**STG:**  Resident will appropriately release feelings of fear, distrust by attending ____________ activity ____________ times per (day, week) by ____________ (date).

**Problems/ Needs:**  Resident refuses to change clothes.

**STG:**  Resident will be clean and well groomed daily over next 90 days.

**STG:**  Resident will agree to change clothes every day over next 90 days.

**Problems/ Needs:**  Resident seems quiet, has had recent roommate change.

**STG:** Resident will agree to talk with (activity director, ___________ other) regarding new roommate by ___________ (date).

**STG:** Resident will talk with new roommate by ___________ (date).

**STG:** Resident will be able to call roommate "friend" by ___________ (date).

**STG:** Resident will talk with ___________ (DON, ADM, ___________ other) regarding desire for roommate change by ___________ (date).

**Approaches:**

1. Schedule visits with resident in private area ___________ times week.

2. Allow resident opportunities to talk about feelings. Be an active listener, make supportive comments such as "I understand."

3. Keep visits friendly and brief until resident seems comfortable — relaxes facial expressions, does not jump/turn away when touched, etc.

4. Encourage resident to verbalize thoughts/feelings.

5. Talk with resident about spending time in communal area.

6. Caution resident during episodes of shortness of breath — remind resident to breathe through diaphragm. Assist resident in breathing by counting slowly in a calm voice.

7. Provide frequent opportunities for resident to stop movement and rest. Position chairs at strategic places in hall, benches on the lawn. Encourage resident to use "rest areas."

8. Encourage participation in discussion group as outlet for "restless" feelings.

9.   Encourage participation in ambulatory exercise as outlet for ("restless" feelings, angry feelings, _____________ other).

10.  Provide therapeutic counseling.

11.  Involve resident in yoga breathing class/Lamaze classes to encourage control over breathing during episodes of shortness of breath.

12.  Remind resident to rest periodically.

13.  Take resident by hand; lead resident to rest area; sit down; invite resident to sit with you.  Chat about current events, resident's interests.

14.  Talk with resident regarding eating habits.  Encourage resident to verbalize feelings.

15.  Provide resident with information regarding what may happen if medications are not taken as order.  Allow resident to make choice.

16.  Respect resident's decision.

17.  Talk with resident regarding change in ADL patterns, allow opportunity to discuss feelings. Encourage resident to verbalize.

18.  Discuss facility policy regarding resident's choice of dress. Encourage resident to wear day clothing during daylight hours.

19.  Provide extra fluids during activities.  Encourage resident to consume.

20.  Talk with resident regarding consequences of "not eating."

21.  Schedule resident for beauty shop/barber appointments.  Encourage resident to go.

22.  Involve resident in feelings support group.  Motivate other residents to assert "peer pressure" as appropriate.

23. HCP team will refer resident for psychiatric evaluation. Request specific guidelines for approaches from psychiatrist for staff to follow.

24. Record approaches when received.

25. Schedule family counseling session with resident.

26. When resident makes sexual advances, inform resident, "That's not why I'm here..." Do not scold. Gently remove resident hand and walk away.

27. Counsel with resident regarding privacy.

28. Remind other residents to close the door to their rooms when not occupied to discourage wandering residents.

29. When resident is observed with another resident's belongings inform resident, "You have Mr. ___________ 's ___________ (tie, shoe, wallet, shirt, ___________ other) by mistake..." Do not accuse them of stealing.  Do not judge.

30. Talk with resident regarding hoarding food/trash in room. Allow time for resident to express self.

31. Inservice nursing staff to take time during care giving activities. Use short, simple phrases.  Explain each activity before beginning.  Continue to talk with resident in calm voice throughout.

32. Talk with resident about need to change clothing on routine basis.

33. Involve resident in the following activities:

    a. ___________ Remotivation group
    b. ___________ Sensory stimulation
    c. ___________ One-on-one visits
    d. ___________ Exercise
    e. ___________ Modified exercise

f. __________ Yoga breathing class
g. __________ Cooking class
h. __________ Crafts
i. __________ Music
j. __________ Sing-a-long
k. __________ Religious services
l. __________ Support group
m. __________ Feelings discussion group
n. __________ Current events
o. __________ Drawing Class
p. __________ Resident Council
q. __________ Other
r. __________ Other

# Activities

Problems that may be triggered in this area include:

1.  new resident, needs to meet other residents and become involved in activities;

2.  new resident, not able to share interests and/or hobby information;

3.  prefers passive activities;

4.  limited involvement in activities because of cognitive decline, grief over loss, declining physical abilities;

5.  exhibits signs of distress, interferes with activity participation;

6.  withdraws to room when invited to participate in activities;

7.  sits on fringe of group, refuses to get involved with others;

8.  expresses thoughts of "…not able to do anymore…;"

9.  has short attention span;

10.  during discussion group tries to talk but thoughts become disorganized;

11.  other residents lose patience with this resident because of disruptive behavior;

12.  bedfast, need one-to-one attention;

13.  needs small group activity with special attention;

14.  states, "I never had time to play when I was healthy, now I don't want to…;"

15.  states, "I don't know how to relax…;"

16. states, "I can't go to the activity because I might wet myself...;"

17. states, "I'm too sick to go to activities...;"

18. states, "If I could hear better, I'd go (to activities) but I can't...;"

19. uses "I'm too tired..." as reason not to attend activities;

20. states, "I'm here for therapy, not to play...;"

21. gets short of breath when asked to play ____________;

22. requires task segmentation to complete craft projects;

23. needs adaptive device to participate in crafts;

24. unable to communicate because of cognitive loss, needs special activities;

25. wishes to learn new skill;

26. has difficulty paying attention when surrounded by other residents;

27. only attends activities if rewarded with prizes and/or refreshments;

28. refuses to attend activities during winter months;

29. refuses activities because "...too far away from my room...;"

30. expresses desire to become resident volunteer;

31. recent change in activity participation;

32. resident is shy, has difficulty making friends;

33. refuses activity participation with certain other residents;

34. active, participates in all activities, then suffers chest pain, shortness of breath, and/or exhaustion;

35. diagnosed with manic depression, needs encouragement to be with others during depressive phase, to be reminded to slow down during manic phase;

36. has tremors which make participation in crafts difficult;

37. expresses desire to go on outings, not able to ambulate independently...

**Care Plan Information The Activity Director May Use:**

**Problems/ Needs:**  New resident, needs to meet other residents and become involved in activities.

**STG:**  Resident will participate in ___________ (activity) ___________ times (week, day) by ___________ (date).

**STG:**  Resident will know names of ___________ (number) of other residents with similar interests by ___________ (date).

**STG:**  Resident will be able to call one other resident "friend" by ___________ (date).

**Problems/ Needs:**  New resident, not able to share interests and/or hobby information.

**STG:**  Resident will agree to talk with activity director ___________ times week and share information regarding interest by ___________ (date).

**STG:**  Resident will choose ___________ (number) of activities of interest per week by ___________ (date).

**STG:**  Resident will agree to attend ___________ (number) of activities ___________ times (week, day) by ___________ (date).

**Problems/
Needs:**   Prefers passive activities participation with others.

**STG:**   Resident will agree to attend _____________ (number) of activities _____________ times per (week, day) by _____________ (date).

**STG:**   Resident will agree to attend one discussion group per _____________ (week, month) and listen by _____________ (date).

**STG:**   Resident will agree to speak during discussion group by _____________ (date).

**Problems/
Needs:**   Limited involvement in activity because of _____________ (cognitive decline, grief over loss of _____________, declining physical abilities, _____________ other.

**STG:**   Resident will agree to attend activities with _____________ (number) of other people _____________ times per (day, week) by _____________ (date).

**STG:**   Resident will attend _____________ (name activity) _____________ times per (day, week) to watch by _____________ (date).

**STG:**   Resident will attend _____________ (number) of activities _____________ times per week by _____________ (date).

**Problems/
Needs:**   Resident exhibits signs of distress, interferers with activity participation.

**STG:**   Resident will agree to talk with activity director, _____________ other) _____________ times per week by _____________ (date).

**STG:** Resident will be able to resume regular activity schedule of ______________ (number) of activities per ______________ (week, month) by ______________ (date).

**Problems/ Needs:** Resident talks about past, makes statements like, "When I was younger, I did all that, now I'm just not interested…"

**STG:** Resident will discuss current interests with activity director by ______________ (date).

**STG:** Resident will be able to say, "I can still do ______________ (name activity)…" by ______________ (date).

**Problems/ Needs:** Resident withdraws to room when invited to participate in activities.

**STG:** Resident will agree to talk with (activity director, ______________ other) regarding reasons for withdrawal by ______________ (date).

**STG:** Resident will agree to sit near door and watch ______________ (name activity) by ______________ (date).

**STG:** Resident will participate in ______________ (activity) by ______________ (date).

**Problems/ Needs:** Resident sits on fringe of group, refuses to get involved with others.

**STG:** Resident will agree to talk with (activity director, ______________ other) by ______________ (date).

**STG:** Resident will agree to talk with ______________ (number) of other residents with similar interests by ______________ (date).

**STG:** Resident will agree to passive participation in ______________ (activity) by ______________ (date).

**STG:** Resident will participate in ___________ (number) of activities by __________ (date).

**Problems/ Needs:** Resident expresses thoughts of "...not able to do anymore..."

**STG:** Resident will agree to talk with (activity director, __________ other) by ___________ (date).

**STG:** Resident will agree to try ___________ (name activity) by ___________ (date).

**STG:** Resident will attend ____________ support group (name group) ____________ times ___________ (week, month) by ____________ (date).

**Problems/ Needs:** Resident refuses inquiries regarding activity interests, states, "Why bother, I can't..."

**STG:** Resident will agree to talk with (activity director, __________ other) by ___________ (date).

**STG:** Resident will agree to try ____________ (name activity) by ___________ (date).

**STG:** Resident will attend ___________ support group ___________ times ___________ (week, month) by ___________ (date).

**STG:** Resident will be able to say, "I can..." by ___________ (date).

**Problems/ Needs:** Resident expresses interests when talking with activity director, but refuses participation and/or attendance to activities.

**STG:** Resident will agree to talk with activity director regarding realistic activity goals by ___________ (date).

**STG:** Resident will agree to try ___________ (name activity) ___________ times per ___________ (day, week, month) by ___________ (date).

**Problems/ Needs:** Resident has difficulty coping with large group situations, seems ___________ (upset, frustrated, angry, ___________ other).

**STG:** Resident will participate in one-to-one activities with (activity director, volunteer, other resident, ___________ other) by ___________ (date).

**STG:** Resident will participate in small group activities ___________ times per ___________ (day, week) by ___________ (date).

**Problems/ Needs:** Resident not able to make choice regarding which activities to attend when offered two at the same time.

**STG:** Resident will be able to make decision ___________ (1 of 5, 2 of 5, 3 of 5, ___________ other) times by ___________ (date).

**STG:** Resident will continue activity___________ times per ___________ (week, month) by ___________ (date).

**Problems/ Needs:** Resident's memory loss problems make participation with other residents difficult.

**STG:** Resident will participate in one-to-one activities with (activity director, volunteer, ___________ other) by ___________ (date).

**STG:** Resident will participate in special activities with ___________ (2, 3, 4,) other residents by ___________ (date).

**STG:** Resident will participate in ___________ (number) small group activities per ___________ (day, week) by ___________ (date).

**Problems/ Needs:** Resident has short attention span, can only sit still for ___________ (number of minutes).

**STG:** Resident will be able to increase attention span from ___________ minutes to ___________ minutes by ___________ (date).

**STG:** Resident will attend ___________ (activity) for ___________ minutes by ___________ (date).

**STG:** Resident will attend ___________ (activity) which fits into his/her short attention span by ___________ (date).

**Problems/ Needs:** During discussion group, resident tries to talk but thoughts become disorganized.

**STG:** Resident will practice conversations with (activity director, ___________ other) ___________ times week by ___________ (date).

**STG:** Resident will be able to attend ___________ (activity) and respond to inclusion with "yes" or "no" answers by ___________ (date).

**STG:** Resident will be able to make simple contributions to discussion group by ___________ (date).

**Problems/ Needs:** Other residents lose patience with resident because of disruptive behavior.

**STG:** Resident will understand his/her ___________ (describe behavior) is annoying to others by ___________ (date).

**STG:**  Resident will attend __________ (number) of small group activities with residents of similar abilities __________ times per (week, month) by ____________ (date).

**Problems/ Needs:**  Resident is bedfast, needs one-to-one attention.

**STG:**  Resident will respond to ______________________________ by ____________ (date).

**STG:**  Resident will talk with ____________ (activity director, volunteer) ____________ times per week by ____________ (date).

**STG:**  Resident will ____________ (open eyes, hold hand, track movement, ____________ other) by ____________ (date).

**STG:**  Resident will do ____________ (name bedside activity) ____________ times week by ____________ (date).

**Problems/ Needs:**  Resident needs small group activity with special attention

**STG:**  Resident will attend ____________ (name small group activity) ____________ times per week by ____________ (date).

**Problems/ Needs:**  Resident states, "I never had time to play when I was healthy, now I don't want to..."

**STG:**  Resident will agree to talk with ____________ (activity director, activity consultant, ______________ other) ____________ times by ____________ (date) regarding leisure counseling.

**STG:**  Resident will agree to try ____________ (name passive activity) ____________ times by ____________ (date).

**STG:** Resident will agree to attend ___________ (activity) by ___________ (date).

**STG:** Resident will participate in ___________ (activity) ___________ times per ___________ (week, month) by ___________ (date).

**Problems/ Needs:** Resident states, "I don't know how to relax…"

**STG:** Resident will agree to one-to-one relaxation activity with___________ (activity director, volunteer, ___________ other) by ___________ (date).

**STG:** Resident will talk about feelings with activity director by ___________ (date).

**STG:** Resident will attend relaxation exercises with other resident ___________ times per week by ___________ (date).

**STG:** Resident will be able to say, "When I need to relax I ___________ (describe what resident does to relax)…," by ___________ (date).

**Problems/ Needs:** Resident states, "I can't go to the activity because I might wet myself…" or "I need to stay close to the bathroom…"

**STG:** Resident will agree to talk with ___________ (social worker, nurse, doctor, ___________ other) regarding bladder control problem by ___________ (date).

**STG:** Resident will take responsibility for self and empty bladder before attending short activity of 30 minutes by ___________ (date).

**STG:** Resident will be able to attend activities of choice by ___________ (date) without fear of embarrassment.

**Problems/
Needs:**  Resident states, "I'm too sick to go to activities…"

**STG:**  Resident will agree to talk with (activity director, _____________ other) _____________ times week by _____________ (date).

**STG:**  Resident will be able to say "okay" to activity attendance by _____________ (date).

**Problems/
Needs:**  Resident states, "I can't go to _____________ (activity) because my _____________ (legs, stomach, head, _____________ other) hurts…"

**STG:**  Resident will agree to talk with (activity director, _____________ other) _____________ times week by _____________ (date).

**STG:**  Resident will attend yoga breathing classes for control of pain _____________ times week by _____________ (date).

**STG:**  Resident will be able to say "okay" to activity attendance by _____________ (date).

**Problems/
Needs:**  Resident states, "If I could hear better, I'd go (to activities) but I can't…"

**STG:**  Resident will agree to hearing evaluation by _____________ (date).

**STG:**  Resident will wear hearing aid daily by _____________ (date).

**STG:**  Resident will take responsibility for self and sit near source of sound during activity _____________ times week by _____________ (date).

**STG:**  Resident will attend _____________ (number) activities _____________ times per week by _____________ (date).

**Problems/ Needs:**  Resident states, "I'm so tired after therapy, I don't want to do anything..."

**STG:**  Resident will understand the value of leisure activities to aid relaxation by _____________ (date).

**STG:**  Resident will agree to one-to-one relaxation activity with _____________ (activity director, volunteer, _____________ other) by _____________ (date).

**STG:**  Resident will attend relaxation exercise by _____________ (date).

**STG:**  Resident will agree to try _____________ (reading, needlework, crossword puzzles, _____________ other) during free time by _____________ (date).

**Problems/ Needs:**  Resident states, "I'm here for therapy, not to play..."

**STG:**  Resident will understand the value of leisure activities and the importance of relaxation by _____________ (date).

**STG:**  Resident will agree to one-on-one leisure counseling _____________ times week by _____________ (date).

**STG:**  Resident will agree to try _____________ (reading, needlework, crossword puzzles, small group activity, _____________ other) by _____________ (date).

**STG:**  Resident will be able to say "okay" to activity participation by _____________ (date).

**Problems/ Needs:**  Resident gets "short of breath" when asked to play _____________ (name of activity), a former favorite leisure pursuit.

**STG:** Resident will agree to talk with activity director regarding feelings by ____________ (date).

**STG:** Resident will remember to relax when playing ____________ (name activity) by ____________ (date).

**STG:** Resident will participate in ____________ (name activity) without fear of "shortness of breath" by ____________ (date).

**Problems/ Needs:** Resident requires task segmentation to complete craft projects.

**STG:** Resident will be able to complete one craft project at each session attended by ____________ (date).

**Problems/ Needs:** Resident needs ____________ adaptive device (name device, example: large crochet hook, C-clamp to hold project, built-up pencil, ____________ other) to participate in crafts.

**STG:** Resident will have ____________ device by ____________ (date).

**STG:** Resident will be able to ____________ (name craft activity) by ____________ (date).

**Problems/ Needs:** Resident unable to communicate because of cognitive loss, needs special activities.

**STG:** Resident will participate in one-to-one activities with ____________ (activity director, volunteer, ____________ other) by ____________ (date).

**STG:** Resident will participate in special activities with ____________ (2, 3, 4,) other residents by ____________ (date).

**STG:** Resident will participate in __________ (number) small group activities per __________ (day, week) by __________ (date).

**Problems/ Needs:** Resident wishes to learn new skill, has expressed desire to __________ (name activity).

**STG:** Resident will learn how to __________ (name activity) by __________ (date).

**STG:** Resident will be able to __________ (name activity) ad lib by __________ (date).

**Problems/ Needs:** Resident has difficulty paying attention when surrounded by other residents, needs individual attention during large group activities.

**STG:** Resident will agree to sit next to __________ (activity director, volunteer, __________ other) during activities by __________ (date).

**Problems/ Needs:** Resident only attends activities if rewarded with prizes and/or refreshments.

**STG:** Resident will agree to try __________ (name activity) for the sheer pleasure of participation by __________ (date).

**STG:** Resident will attend __________ (number) activities per __________ (week, month) without reward of prize or refreshments by __________ (date).

**STG:** Resident's rights will be respected by staff.

**Problems/ Needs:** Resident refuses to attend activities during winter months, states, "It's too cold to do anything..."

**STG:**  Resident will agree to talk with (activity director, ___________ other) ___________ times week by ___________ (date).

**STG:**  Resident will discuss feelings behind excuse by ___________ (date).

**STG:**  Resident will take responsibility for self and wear sweater and/or shawl when feeling cold by ___________ (date).

**STG:**  Resident will attend ___________ (activity) ___________ times per week by ___________ (date).

**Problems/ Needs:**  Resident says, "I'd go to activities, but they are so far away from my room..."

**STG:**  Resident will agree to assistance of ___________ (wheel-chair ride to and from activity, nurse assistant's arm to lean on ___________ other) by ___________ (date).

**STG:**  Resident will agree to try ___________ activity in dining room before noon meal ___________ times week by ___________ (date).

**STG:**  Resident will talk with ___________ (SW, DON, ADM,) regarding room change closer to activity area by ___________ (date).

**STG:**  Resident will agree to in-room activity of ___________ (name activity) by ___________ (date).

**Problems/ Needs:**  Resident expresses desire to become resident volunteer, states, "I'd like to do something for others..."

**STG:**  Resident will agree to ___________ (become hostess at parties, deliver resident mail, assist with mailing for local charity, ___________ other) by ___________ (date).

**STG:** Resident will agree to report volunteer hours to activity director each day by ___________ (date).

**Problems/ Needs:** Resident was active in activities of choice until recently when ___________ (describe what is the suspected cause of problem).

**STG:** Resident will agree to talk with (activity director, ___________ other) ___________ times week by ___________ (date).

**STG:** Resident will be able to work through problem and become active in activities ___________ times (day, week) by ___________ (date).

**Problems/ Needs:** Resident is shy, has difficulty making friends.

**STG:** Resident will agree to allow (activity director, ___________ other) to introduce him/her to other resident by ___________ (date).

**STG:** Resident will respond to friendly advances of other residents by talking with ___________ (number) of other residents each day by ___________ (date).

**STG:** Resident will be able to say, "I have a friend..." by ___________ (date).

**Problems/ Needs:** Resident states, "I'll go to this activity if ___________ (other female resident, other male resident—do not use other resident's name) doesn't go..."

**STG:** Resident will agree to talk with (activity director, ___________ other) regarding feelings by ___________ (date).

**STG:** Resident will say "okay" to activities without reservations by ___________ (date).

**Problems/ Needs:**  Resident is active, participates in all activities offered, then suffers from ___________ (chest pains, shortness of breath, exhaustion, ___________ other).

**STG:**  Resident will take responsibility for self and rest for ___________ (number) of ___________ (minutes, hours) after each activity by ___________ (date).

**Problems/ Needs:**  Resident diagnosed with manic depression (bi-polar depression) needs ___________ (much encouragement to be with others during depression phase, to be reminded to slow down during manic phase).

**STG:**  Resident will be able to ___________ (come out of room for ___________ number minutes each day, talk with ___________ number people each day, ___________ other) during depressed phase.

**STG:**  Resident will rest for ___________ (number) ___________ (minutes, hours) after each activity by ___________ (date).

**Problems/ Needs:**  Resident wants to (write, draw, sew, crochet, ___________ other) but gets frustrated when tremors increase and prevent this activity.

**STG:**  Resident will talk with (activity director, ___________ other) ___________ regarding feelings as needed by ___________ (date).

**STG:**  Resident will remember to relax by ___________ (doing deep breathing exercises, practicing yoga breathing techniques, counting slowly, ___________ other) when tremors occur by ___________ (date).

**Problems/ Needs:**  Resident expresses desire to go on outings, but not able to ambulate independently.

**STG:** Resident will agree to assistance of ___________ (one-to-one volunteer, use of walker, use of wheelchair, ___________ other) during outings away from facility ___________ times month by ___________ (date).

## Approaches:

1.  Take resident on tour of facility; introduce resident to staff and other residents.

2.  Continually use resident's full name, use full name of others in grouping with residents to reinforce memory of other resident's names.

3.  Continually introduce staff and self to resident; use names often to assist resident in remembering.

4.  Introduce resident to other residents of similar interests; encourage conversation.

5.  Encourage resident to explore facility on his/her own.

6.  Encourage resident to visit with other residents.

7.  Introduce resident to roommate, use name often to assist resident in remembering.

8.  Visit with resident individually. Discuss activities offered. Encourage resident to show interest by ___________ (discussing those of interest, nodding head when activity of interest is mentioned, ___________ other).

9.  Review resident rights with new resident, repeat again a few weeks later. Ask questions of resident to determine whether or not resident understands.

10. Invite resident to assist in planning activities of interest to resident.

11.  Ask resident for ideas regarding program planning; use resident's ideas if feasible, if not explain why not to resident and request further ideas.

12.  Involve resident in the following activities:

    a.  __________  New resident discussion group
    b.  __________  Support Group
    c.  __________  Movies
    d.  __________  Entertainments
    e.  __________  Beauty shop/barbershop
    f.  __________  Resident Council
    g.  __________  Exercise
    h.  __________  Other

13.  Involve resident in the following passive activities:

    a.  __________  Movies
    b.  __________  Parties
    c.  __________  Entertainments
    d.  __________  Lecture series
    e.  __________  Demonstration classes
    f.  __________  Beauty shop/barber shop
    g.  __________  Manicures
    h.  __________  Other

14.  Evaluate resident's abilities to participate in small group activities for cognitively impaired resident.

15.  Provide small group activities with 2 or 3 residents such as:

    a.  __________  Special exercise
    b.  __________  Special crafts
    c.  __________  Music/movement
    d.  __________  Walks around building
    e.  __________  Reminiscence therapy
    f.  __________  Remotivation group
    g.  __________  Sensory stimulation
    h.  __________  Memory classes

i. __________ "Win" (special bingo)
j. __________ Parties
k. __________ Validation therapy
l. __________ Sing-a-longs
m. __________ Other

16. HCP team will evaluate resident for need of therapeutic counseling.

17. Refer to __________ for counseling sessions __________ times per (week, month).

18. Provide resident with opportunities to talk about feelings; provide feedback to social worker.

19. Invite resident to attend:

a. __________ Arthritis support group
b. __________ Stroke group
c. __________ Diabetes support group
d. __________ Feelings discussion group
e. __________ Current events
f. __________ Moderate exercise
g. __________ Yoga breathing classes
h. __________ Other

20. Encourage other residents in the group to be supportive of resident when he/she makes positive statements about himself/herself.

21. Encourage use of peer pressure to confront resident when making self-depreciating comments about self.

22. Schedule regular appointments at beauty shop/barber shop __________ times month; encourage resident to keep appointments.

23. Reward appropriate behavior with much praise; ignore negative behavior.

24. Talk with resident about "watching" activities for a few minutes before deciding whether or not to leave.

25. Do not pressure resident, but be warm and friendly while observing activities.

26. Let resident know he may leave activity at any time, encourage resident to give activity a "try."

27. Allow the resident to "sit and watch" for a few times before gently bringing him/her into group. Do not pressure participation. Involve resident at first by asking "yes" or "no" type questions.

28. Visit with resident following activity; offer verbal praise for __________ (observing, responding to superficial questions, talking/participating in activity, __________ other).

29. Schedule one-to-one visits with resident to review activity interests/needs. Encourage resident to share information.

30. Review goal setting with resident. Encourage resident to set his/her own activity goals.

31. Schedule individual sessions with resident to work on decision making.

32. Encourage resident to make simple choices.

33. Reward decisions with praise.

34. Encourage resident to "stick with decision" by offering praise.

35. Schedule bedside visits with resident __________ times per __________ (week, day).

36. Provide the following bedside activities:

    a. __________ Mobiles
    b. __________ Music

c.  __________  Puzzles
d.  __________  Reading
e.  __________  Volunteer visits
f.  __________  Colorful pictures
g.  __________  Therapeutic counseling
h.  __________  Sensory stimulation
i.  __________  Bird feeder outside window
j.  __________  One-on-one discussion of current events
k.  __________  Newspaper
l.  __________  Other residents visiting in small groups
m.  __________  Crafts
n.  __________  Bed exercise to increase circulation
o.  __________  Other

37.  Schedule leisure counseling sessions for resident.  Explore leisure interests.  Evaluate resident physical abilities, environmental needs for adjustment, emotional needs to use free time.

38.  Plan class for resident to learn how to play the following games:

a.  __________  Dominoes
b.  __________  Cards
c.  __________  Checkers
d.  __________  Darts
e.  __________  Scrabble
f.  __________  Scatagories
g.  __________  Horseshoes
h.  __________  Bowling
i.  __________  Pool/billiards
j.  __________  Table hockey
k.  __________  Trivia
l.  __________  Monopoly
m.  __________  Table tennis
n.  __________  Brain teasers
o.  __________  Crossword puzzles
p.  __________  "Search-a-word"
q.  __________  "Find the difference"
r.  __________  Other

39.  Involve resident in realization classes with other residents.

40.  Encourage residents to "go to the bathroom" just prior to activity beginning.  Remind to go again at the end of the activity.

41.  Investigate resident's complaints of pain in __________ (legs, stomach, head, __________ other).

42.  Encourage resident to talk with nurse regarding physical complaints.  Inform nurse of resident's complaints.

43.  Provide opportunities for resident to discuss feelings/emotions.

44.  Refer to social worker for therapeutic counseling sessions for resident with many somatic complaints.

45.  Provide resident with calendar of events; encourage resident to pick one activity/event a week to attend.  Encourage follow through on the resident's part.

46.  Involve resident in yoga breathing classes for control of pain.

47.  Invite resident to sit near activity leader to better __________ (see, hear).

48.  Break instructions down into short simple phrases.  Allow time for resident to complete one step before giving the next step.

49.  Evaluate resident for use of the following adaptive device:

    a.  __________  C-clamp
    b.  __________  Built-up pencil
    c.  __________  Universal cuff
    d.  __________  Built-up paint brush
    e.  __________  Extra large crochet hook, knitting needles
    f.  __________  Other

50.  Include resident in following activities:

for refreshments:
a.  __________  Parties
b.  __________  Entertainment
c.  __________  Coffee social
d.  __________  Happy hour
e.  __________  Other

for prizes:
a.  __________  Bingo
b.  __________  Games
c.  __________  Other

51.  Talk with resident regarding need for warm clothes.  Evaluate resident's response to "winter months."

52.  Refer to social worker for therapeutic counseling as needed.

53.  Talk with resident about using a wheelchair to go to and from activity area if more than 50 feet.  Provide chair if needed.

54.  Talk with resident about use of __________ (assistance of nursing assistant, walker, cane, __________ other).  Provide same if needed.

55.  Encourage resident to make room change request if desires to be closer to activity action.

56.  Involve resident in the following resident-volunteer program:

a.  __________  Assist serving refreshments at parties.
b.  __________  Pass out bingo equipment to other residents.
c.  __________  Deliver mail to residents in afternoon.
d.  __________  Visit with ______ number of bedfast residents to read/chat.
e.  __________  Address/stuff envelopes for __________ charity.
f.  __________  Assist ______ number of other residents to remember to go to activity.

g.    _________ Participate on newspaper.
h.    _________ Run for office in Resident Council.
i.    _________ Work on decoration committee.
j.    _________ Work on welcome committee.
k.    _________ Work on birthday committee.
l.    _________ Work on hospital committee.
m.    _________ Other

57. Schedule one-to-one visit with resident to discuss feelings behind comments made regarding other residents. Encourage resident to _________ (talk with other residents and work out reasonable solution to problem, avoid other residents, _________ other).

58. Remind resident to rest as needed throughout day. Encourage actual rest in bed for _________ (minutes, hours) per day.

59. Encourage resident to spend _________ number (minutes, hours) out of room in social area.

60. Invite resident to go on quiet walks for 10-20 minutes out of doors.

61. Provide resident with friendly one-to-one visits to chat about current events.

62. Include resident in one of the following classes to aid relaxation:

a.    _________ Yoga breathing classes
b.    _________ Relaxation/imagery class
c.    _________ Modified exercise
d.    _________ Other

# Falls

Problems that may be triggered in this area include:

1.   at risk for falls because of medication;

2.   at risk for falls because of prosthesis poorly fitting;

3.   at risk for falls due to inability to control body movement;

4.   at risk for falls due to inability to transfer self;

5.   at risk for falls due to acute episodes of weakness;

6.   at risk for falls due to poor vision...

**Care Plan Information The Activity Director May Use:**

(Note:  As in the area of ADL's the nurse may be the person citing problems and goals in this area. The Activity Director may wish to add Approaches.)

**Approaches:**

1.   Observe arrangement of activity room for hazards, rearrange. Alert resident to changes.

2.   Educate resident in locating different areas of building/architectural barriers.

3.   Encourage resident to use available hearing to determine obstacles that may present hazards.

4.   Caution resident to be careful when moving from seated position to standing.  Encourage resident to count to five slowly before beginning to walk.

5.   Report any falls during activities to nursing staff immediately. Do not move resident, wait for the licensed nurse to check resident first before attempting to help resident up off the floor.

# Oral/Nutritional Status

Problems that may be triggered in this area include:

1. unable to chew;

2. complains of pain in mouth when chewing;

3. ill-fitting dentures/bridges;

4. forgets to chew food, potential for choking, potential for weight loss;

5. difficulty swallowing;

6. coughs during meal service or when drinking, potential for aspiration and/or choking;

7. holds food in mouth;

8. spills food from mouth because of excessive drooling;

9. dryness of mouth, not able to swallow;

10. weight loss;

11. weight gain;

12. below ideal body weight;

13. above ideal body weight;

14. complains about taste of food;

15. complains about bad taste in mouth;

16. complains of hunger;

17. forgets he/she has eaten;

18.  has history of dehydration;

19.  poor intake of fluid, at risk for dehydration;

20.  complains, "I'm never full, I always feel hungry...;"

21.  keeps snacks in room, refuses food at mealtime;

22.  has small appetite;

23.  refuses to eat;

24.  refuses to follow physician's diet order;

25.  becomes combative, hostile, angry, abusive when served diet according to physician's diet order;

26.  family brings food in conflict with physician's diet order;

27.  disruptive behavior in dining room;

28.  refuses to dress appropriately for meals;

29.  takes food from other residents at table;

30.  throws food;

31.  spits on floor;

32.  throws dishes;

33.  abnormal lab values;

34.  shows progressive weight loss while consuming more than 1800-2000 calories each day;

35.  wishes to feed self, has difficulty getting food on utensil, drops food;

36.  needs tube feeding;

37. needs increased caloric intake due to constant motion, constant walking, tardive dyskinesia, draining wound, burns, recent long bone/hip fracture, dialysis, or chemotherapy;

38. unable to swallow due to dysphagia, neuro-muscular deterioration, confusion, or persistent vegetative state;

39. dislodges NG tube, G tube, nasoduodenal tube, jejunostomy tube by pulling at tube, constant motion in bed, or exaggerated movement;

40. does not tolerate tube feedings;

41. has advanced directive "No tube feedings," not able/willing to eat...

**Care Plan Information The Activity Director May Use:**

(Note: Problems and goals in this area will probably be identified either by the consultant dietitian, the dietary manager, or the nurse. The Activity Director's input would be included in the approaches to problems cited.)

**Approaches:**

1. Refer to dentist for evaluation and treatment.

2. Provide resident with unhurried atmosphere for meals and during refreshments at activities.

3. Remind resident (to chew, to eat, to chew more slowly, to slow down, __________ other).

4. Supervise resident closely during meals and refreshments during activities.

5. Evaluate psychosocial needs, emotional status which may cause feelings of hunger.

6.  Serve ice cream, gelatins, puddings, _________ times daily and/ or during activities.

7.  Remind resident to drink water.

8.  Offer water to resident each time room is entered.

9.  Offer fluids during activity participation.

10.  Evaluate for mood or cognitive status change.

11.  Evaluate resident ability to communicate food needs, food preferences.

12.  Counsel with resident regarding feelings, offer appropriate outlets for negative feelings.

13.  Encourage resident to discuss feelings; discourage food throwing by ignoring behavior.

14.  Assist dietary manager in talking with family regarding resident's diet as ordered by physician. Request family only bring allowed items.

15.  Counsel with resident regarding facility policy on _________ (appropriate dress for meal service, acceptable behavior at the table, _________ other).

16.  Inform dietary manager regarding refreshments consumed during activities.

17.  Talk with resident/family about feelings regarding tube feedings.

18.  Offer emotional support.

# Oral and Dental

Problems that may be triggered in this area include:

1.   complains of mouth pain;

2.   shows signs that he/she may be experiencing mouth pain, i.e., refusing to chew and/or refusing to drink hot or cold liquids;

3.   poor oral hygiene, not able to brush own teeth;

4.   pockets food in mouth;

5.   does not, not able to adequately clean teeth/dentures;

6.   has multiple dental caries;

7.   has broken teeth;

8.   has missing teeth - needs dental evaluation;

9.   has lost denture/bridge;

10.   dentures/bridge are broken/poorly fitting;

11.   refuses to wear dentures;

12.   mouth coated with film; lips are dry, sticky;

13.   has swollen, inflamed gums;

14.   ulcers/rashes on gums;

15.   bleeding gums…

**Care Plan Information The Activity Director May Use:**

**Problems/ Needs:** Resident complains of mouth pain; shows signs that he/ she may be experiencing mouth pain __________ (refusing to chew, refusing to drink hot or cold liquids, __________ other).

**STG:** Mouth pain will clear, resident will be able to eat without discomfort by __________ (date).

**STG:** Dental evaluation will occur by __________ (date).

**Problems/ Needs:** Resident has multiple dental caries; has broken teeth; missing teeth — needs dental evaluation.

**STG:** Resident will agree to see dentist by __________ (date).

**STG:** Dental evaluation will occur by __________ (date).

**STG:** Resident will be free of pain from __________ (dental caries, broken teeth, missing teeth) by __________ (date).

**Problems/ Needs:** Resident has lost denture/bridge; resident's dentures/ bridge are lost/broken/poorly fitting.

**STG:** Dentures/bridge will be replaced/repaired by __________ (date).

**STG:** Resident will be able to chew without choking by __________ (date).

**Problems/ Needs:** Resident has swollen, inflamed gums; ulcers/rashes on gums; bleeding gums.

**STG:** __________ (record problem condition) will clear by __________ (date).

**STG:** Dental evaluation will occur by __________ (date).

**Approaches:**

1. Provide resident with toothbrush and toothpaste.  Encourage resident to brush per self.

2. Remind resident to brush teeth after __________ (each meal, daily, __________ other).

3. Schedule dental exam/evaluation.

4. Provide necessary transportation to dentist.

5. Offer fluids throughout the day and when refreshments are served.

6. Seek financial assistance from __________ (family, insurance, __________ other) to provide appropriate dental care.

# Pressure Sores

Problems that may be triggered in this area include:

1.  at risk for pressure sores due to impaired mobility, bedfast, hemiplegia, paraplegia, quadriplegia, bowel or bladder incontinence, decreased circulation, elevated blood sugar, recent fracture, weight loss, past history of pressure sores, loss of sensitivity to pain and discomfort, daily use of antipsychotics or antidepressants, daily use of restraints, excessive diarrhea, systemic infection, end stage renal disease, steroid therapy, radiation therapy, chemotherapy, renal dialysis, peritoneal dialysis, underweight, or overweight;

2.  resident has pressure sore stage _______, _______ cm, ___________ (location).

**Care Plan Information The Activity Director May Use:**

(Note: Problems and goals for skin integrity will be cited by the nurse with input from the Activity Director, the dietitian and others in the area of approaches.)

**Approaches:**

1.  Provide exercise program for bedfast.

2.  Use music to stimulate movement.

3.  Provide the following bedside activities:

    a.  _________ Reading
    b.  _________ Puzzles
    c.  _________ Taped music
    d.  _________ Volunteer visits
    e.  _________ Mobiles
    f.  _________ Colorful pictures
    g.  _________ Sensory stimulation

h. __________ Bird feeder outside window
i. __________ One-to-one discussion of current events
j. __________ Visiting residents in small group discussion
k. __________ Crafts
l. __________ Bed exercise to increase circulation
n. __________ Other

# Psychotropic Drug Use

Problems that may be triggered in this area include:

1. episodes of low blood pressure due to psychotropic medications;

2. episodes of dizziness due to psychotropic medications;

3. episodes of lost consciousness due to psychotropic medications;

4. episodes of recurrent falls due to psychotropic medication;

5. has difficulty walking, shuffles feet, unable to walk straight due to psychotropic medications;

6. unable to turn self in bed due to psychotropic medications;

7. periods of constant, restless movement/motor agitation due to psychotropic medications;

8. episodes of inappropriate behavior due to psychotropic medication use;

9. episodes of hallucinations due to psychotropic medications;

10. episodes of constipation due to psychotropic medications;

11. episodes of fecal impactions due to psychotropic medication use;

12. experiences urinary retention due to use of psychotropic medications;

13. experiences episodes of edema due to use of psychotropic medications...

**Care Plan Information The Activity Director May Use:**

(Note:  Problems and goals will be set by nursing.  The Activity Director's input will be in the area of approaches.)

**Approaches:**

1.  Observe for dry mouth and report to nursing.

2.  Observe for tremors and report to nursing.

3.  Observe for lip smacking and report to nursing.

4.  Observe for rapid movement of tongue and report to nursing.

5.  Observe for drowsiness and report to nursing.

6.  Observe for blurred vision and report to nursing.

7.  Observe for fever and report to nursing.

8.  Observe for lack of perspiration and report to nursing.

9.  Encourage liquid refreshments during activities.

10. Encourage resident to come out of room for:

| | | |
|---|---|---|
| a. | _________ | Parties |
| b. | _________ | Entertainments |
| c. | _________ | Discussion group |
| d. | _________ | Remotivation therapy |
| e. | _________ | Support group |
| f. | _________ | Counseling sessions |
| g. | _________ | Beauty shop |
| h. | _________ | Arts and crafts |
| i. | _________ | Religious services |
| j. | _________ | Games |
| k. | _________ | Drama club |
| l. | _________ | Sing-a-longs |
| m. | _________ | Exercise class |
| n. | _________ | Other |
| o. | _________ | Other |

# Physical Restraints

Problems that may be triggered in this area include:

1. may have increase in inappropriate behavior due to use of physical restraints, i.e., kicking, biting, scratching, screaming, or yelling;

2. experiences episodes of constipation/chronic constipation due to use of physical restraints;

3. experiences urinary and/or fecal incontinence due to use of physical restraints;

4. has pressure sores due to use of physical restraints;

5. experiences loss of muscle tone due to use of physical restraints;

6. experiences loss of independent mobility due to use of physical restraints;

7. exhibits increased agitation due to use of physical restraints;

8. exhibits loss of balance due to use of physical restraints;

9. exhibits symptoms of withdrawal and/or excessive sadness due to use of physical restraints;

10. has reduced social contacts due to use of physical restraints;

11. may be at risk for additional physical and/or social-emotional problems due to use of physical restraints…

**Care Plan Information The Activity Director May Use:**

**Problems/**   May have increase in inappropriate behavior due to use
**Needs:**   of physical restraints. Resident exhibits __________ (kicking, biting, scratching, screaming, yelling, __________ other).

**STG:** Episodes of ___________ (kicking, biting, scratching, screaming, yelling ___________ other) will be reduced from ___________ (number times per day, week) to ___________ (number times per day, week) by ___________ (date).

**STG:** Resident will be free of ___________ by ___________ (date).

**Problems/ Needs:** Resident exhibits increased agitation due to use of physical restraints.

**STG:** Resident will be calm daily by ___________ (date).

**Problems/ Needs:** Resident exhibits symptoms of withdrawal and/or excessive sadness due to use of physical restraints.

**STG:** Resident will return to normal mood of ___________ (describe normal mood) by ___________ (date).

**STG:** Resident will interact with ___________ (number of others) ___________ times per day by ___________ (date).

**Problems/ Needs:** Resident has reduced social contact due to use of physical restraints.

**STG:** Resident will interact with ___________ (number of others) ___________ times per day by ___________ (date).

**STG:** Resident will be able to interact ad lib by ___________ (date).

**Problems/ Needs:** Resident may be at risk for additional social-emotional problems due to use of physical restraints.

**STG:** Resident will be free of social-emotional complications of restrictive restraints daily over the next 90 days.

**Approaches:**

1.  HCP team will evaluate for use of ___________ restrictive restraint; consider use of ___________ (pillows, pads, removable lap trays, floor mats, controlled activity area, ___________ other).

2.  Consult OTR/LPT for development of less restrictive environmental restraint such as special wheelchair, walkers, pads, etc.

3.  Observe for:

    a. ___________ Increased inappropriate behavior
    b. ___________ Increased agitation
    c. ___________ Loss of balance
    d. ___________ Symptoms of withdrawal or excessive sadness
    e. ___________ Reduced social contact

4.  Be observant to resident's behavior, attempt to interpret same to staff.

5.  Include resident in the following activities:

    a. ___________ Modified exercise
    b. ___________ Sing-a-long
    c. ___________ Religious services
    d. ___________ Discussion groups
    e. ___________ Games
    f. ___________ Arts and crafts
    g. ___________ Remotivation groups
    h. ___________ Counseling sessions
    i. ___________ Volunteer visits
    j. ___________ Other
    k. ___________ Other

# Acquired Immune Deficiency Syndrome (AIDS)

Problems often associated with AIDS may include:

1.   Susceptible to secondary infections such as colds, flu, etc.;

2.   periodic episodes of elevated temperature;

3.   lethargic;

4.   often tires easily;

5.   difficulty walking;

6.   persistent diarrhea;

7.   severe weight loss;

8.   anorexia;

9.   low weight for height;

10.  loss of appetite;

11.  prone to skin breakdown;

12.  skin lesions,

13.  Kaposi's Sarcoma ( a form of skin cancer);

14.  prone to pneumonia;

15.  shortness of breath;

16.  difficulty breathing;

17.  gradual loss of motor function;

18.  gradual loss of speech;

19.  difficulty speaking;

20.  speech slurred, slow;

21.  grief over loss of self image;

22.  loss of close friends;

23.  loss of significant others;

24.  age difference with other residents;

25.  loses train of thought;

26.  disoriented;

27.  depression;

28.  fear of dying;

29.  increasing loss of ability to care for self;

30.  distress in limitation of activities;

31.  semi-comatose

**Care Plan Information The Activity Director Could Use:**

**Problems/** Lethargic; often tires easily.
  **Needs:**

    **STG:**  Resident will rest ______________ (minutes, hours) daily.

    **STG:**  Resident will be able to complete __________ (task, activity by ____________ (date).

**Problems/** Severe weight loss; loss of appetite.
  **Needs:**

    **STG:**  Resident will consume refreshments (within limits of his/her diet) during activities by ____________ (date).

**Problems/ Needs:** Shortness of breath; difficulty breathing.

**STG:** Resident will be able to sing ____________ (number) of songs by ____________ (date).

**STG:** Resident will participate in ____________ (activity) by ____________ (date).

**Problems/ Needs:** Gradual loss of motor function; difficulty walking; muscle spasms; distress over loss of ability to care for self.

**STG:** Resident will be able to (continue feeding self, groom hair, brush teeth, ____________ other) by ____________ (date).

**STG:** Resident will understand disease process by ____________ (date).

**STG:** Resident will participate in group discussion by ____________ (date).

**Problems/ Needs:** Gradual loss of speech; difficulty speaking; speech slurred, slow.

**STG:** Resident will be able to communicate needs by ________ (date).

**STG:** Resident will be able to continue speaking.

**STG:** Resident will be able to use communication board by ____________ (date).

**Problems/ Needs:** Grief over loss of self image; loss of close friends; decreased self esteem; loss of significant other; depressed; fear of dying

**STG:** Resident will verbalize feelings as they occur.

**STG:**  Resident will participate in AIDS support group by ___________ (date).

**STG:**  Resident will talk with ___________ (activity director, social worker, clergy, other) by ____________ (date).

**STG:**  Resident will participate in group discussion for support and positive feelings about self and others by ___________ (date).

**Problems/ Needs:**  Confusion; disoriented; difficulty maintaining train of thought; easily frustrated.

**STG:**  Resident will be able to complete sentences by ____________ (date).

**STG:**  Resident will be able to remember ___________ by ____________ (date).

**STG:**  Resident will attend ___________ (activity) by _________ (date).

**Problems/ Needs:**  Semi-comatose; bedfast

**STG:**  Resident will respond to ____________ by ____________ (date).

**STG:**  Resident will squeeze hand of activity director during one-on-one visits by ____________ (date).

**STG:**  Resident will open eyes during one-on-one visits by ____________ (date).

**STG:**  Resident will look at activity director during one-on-one visits by ____________ (date).

**STG:**  Resident will ___________ (blink eyes, smile, other) during one-on-one visits by ____________ (date).

5. **STG:** Resident will be able to communicate needs through use of __________ (eye contact, communication board, cards, pad and pencil, other) by __________ (date).

**Problems/ Needs:** Inability to cope with age difference with other residents; low socialization.

**STG:** Resident will participate in group discussion with other residents with similar interests __________ (number) times __________ (week, month).

**STG:** Resident will verbalize feelings with activity director __________ (number) times week by __________ (date).

**STG:** Resident will agree to talk with __________ (number) of __________ (residents, staff, volunteers) per day by __________ (date).

**STG:** Resident will spend __________ (amount of time) out of room daily by __________ (date).

## Approaches:

1. Evaluate for less strenuous activities; leisure counseling.

2. Encourage participation in activities that allow minimum of physical participation such as sing-a-long, parties, bingo, entertainments, (other).

3. Provide resident with materials for in-room activities, i.e. reading, painting, jig saw puzzles, other.

4. Encourage participation in activities that foster lung expansion such as sing-a-long, voice exercise, yoga breathing, other, with physician's consent.

5. Serve refreshments from parties, coffee, juice cart, __________ (times) a week.

6.   Work with resident one-on-one on self feeding, combing/brushing hair, brushing teeth, other.  Provide self-help device.

7.   Involve resident in ADL training group for __________ (type of training).

8.   Involve resident in AIDS support group __________ (times) __________ (week, month).

9.   Include resident in feelings group discussions.

10.  Provide resident with communication board; teach how to use.

11.  Make arrangements for speech therapy evaluation with physician's order.

12.  Visit with resident one-on-one, provide opportunities to talk about feelings; offer support; help resident to identify feelings.

13.  Make arrangements for counseling from appropriate party, i.e. social worker familiar with AIDS victims, clergy, psychiatrist, psychologist, other.

14.  Visit with resident for individual sensory stimulation program, work on __________ (activity).

15.  Visit with resident one-on-one, monitor responses to visits. Talk about current events, activities of interest to resident such as __________ (interest).

16.  Provide volunteers to visit for socialization.

17.  Encourage resident to stay __________ (number) minutes in the __________ (activity room, living room, TV room, other).

18.  Observe proper hand washing techniques to prevent cross contamination; maintain equipment in proper fashion according to infection control procedures of facility.

# Alcoholism

Problems often associated with the disease Alcoholism include:

1.   prone to convulsions;

2.   susceptible to infections;

3.   loss of memory;

4.   prone to fluid retention and edema;

5.   prone to peptic ulcers;

6.   excessive intake of tranquilizers

7.   possible liver disorder;

8.   skin hemorrhages;

9.   loss of appetite;

10.  anorexia;

11.  malnutrition;

12.  nausea;

13.  electrolyte imbalance;

14.  manipulation of others;

15.  often hostile;

16.  sometimes aggressive;

17.  abusive of others;

18.  curses frequently;

19.  "sneaky" about ingestion of alcohol;

20.  often depressed;

21.  cries easily;

22.  hallucinates;

23.  exhibits poor hygiene…

## Care Plan Information The Activity Director Could Use:

**Problems/ Needs:**  Loss of memory; difficulty remembering people, places, time; cannot remember the time of specific activities; cannot find his/her room, etc.

**STG:**  Resident will be able to remember _____________ by _____________ (date).

**Problems/ Needs:**  Manipulative of others; will not ask for wants directly, uses many phrases such as "If only we could," or "I wish I had…," etc.

**STG:**  Resident will ask for wants/desires directly by _____________ (date).

**STG:**  Resident will be aware of manipulative behavior and accept confrontation by _____________ (date).

**Problems/ Needs:**  Often hostile; sometimes acts aggressively towards staff or other residents; abusive toward others; curses frequently when does not get his/her way; strikes out at others; abusive towards roommate; etc.

**STG:**  Resident will agree to participate in feelings group by _____________ (date).

**STG:**  Resident will verbally express self in a socially acceptable manner when angry, hostile, aggressive, depressed, etc. by _____________ (date).

**STG:** Resident will agree to express feelings with staff as necessary.

**STG:** Resident will not harm self or others.

**Problems/ Needs:** Often depressed; makes many statements regarding suicide; cries easily for no apparent reason; hallucinates; complains of many physical problems as excuse not to participate in activities; etc.

**STG:** Resident will agree to discuss feelings with __________ (activity director, social worker, counselor) by __________ (date).

**STG:** Resident will have increased self esteem as is evidenced by participation in __________ (beauty shop/barber shop, good grooming class, manicures, etc.) __________ (number) times weekly by __________ (date).

**STG:** Resident will participate in feelings discussion group __________ (number) times weekly by __________ (date).

**STG:** Resident will participate in __________ (number) of activities weekly by __________ (date).

**Problems/ Needs:** Exhibits poor hygiene; needs new clothing because of recent weight gain; will not shave, brush teeth, comb hair; refuses bath; etc.

**STG:** Resident will continue to perform the following tasks for self daily: brush hair, teeth, dress, bathe, shave, other by __________ (date).

**STG:** Resident will participate in good grooming class on __________ (date).

**STG:** Resident will shop for new clothes with volunteer, staff by __________ (date).

**STG:**  Resident will be clean and well groomed daily.

**STG:**  Resident will accept clothing donation from volunteers by ___________ (date).

**Approaches:**

1.  One-on-one to work on remembering ___________.

2.  Involve resident in current events discussion group on ___________ (day).

3.  Be consistent in all activities with resident; do not scold or reprimand.

4.  Set schedule, remind resident matter of factly, encourage staff to do likewise.

5.  Confront abusive or otherwise socially unacceptable behavior as such; encourage resident to verbalize feelings instead of acting out.

6.  Talk with family, elicit their help in control of negative behavior.

7.  One-on-one consultation with resident regarding behavior, let resident know how others see him/her.

8.  Encourage proper grooming by verbally rewarding resident for maintaining self in socially acceptable manner.

9.  Schedule for beauty/barber shop.

10.  Involve resident in group discussion ___________ (number) times weekly on ___________ (days).

11.  Involve resident in AA meetings, provide transportation if necessary.

12.  Be firm, calm, and forceful in all communications with resident.

13. Encourage resident to interact with other residents.

14. Involve resident in the following activities:

    a. __________ Group discussions
    b. __________ Residents Council
    c. __________ Arts and crafts
    d. __________ Current events
    e. __________ Religious services
    f. __________ Exercise and/or movement
    g. __________ Entertainments
    h. __________ Parties - do not serve alcoholic beverages
    i. __________ Awareness groups
    j. __________ Games, bingo, cards, dominoes
    k. __________ Outside excursions and/or outings
    l. __________ Nature walks
    m. __________ Other
    n. __________ Other

# Alzheimer's Disease, Senile Dementia, OBS, CBS

Problems often associated with the diseases Alzheimer's, Senile Dementia, Organic Brain Syndrome, and Chronic Brain Syndrome include:

1.  inability to understand others;

2.  overtly occupied with self;

3.  difficulty making decisions;

4.  loses train of thought easily;

5.  short attention span;

6.  unable to perform activities of daily living for self;

7.  easily frustrated;

8.  hostile toward others

9.  overtly dependent on others;

10.  wanders around, needs constant supervision;

11.  unable/difficulty identifying others;

12.  decreased interaction with others;

13.  often "scapegoated" by others;

14.  exhibits fear when touched...

**Care Plan Information The Activity Director Could Use:**

**Problems/ Need:** Inability to understand others; unable to hold conversation with others; loses train of thought easily; short attention span; decreased interaction with others; etc.

**STG:** Resident will be able to answer simple "yes" or "no" type questions by ___________ (date).

**STG:** Resident will be able to follow simple directions by ___________ (date).

**STG:** Resident will be able to answer simple questions by ___________ (date).

**STG:** Resident will participate in conversation with activity director, staff, other resident by ___________ (date).

**STG:** Resident will initiate conversation with one other person daily by ___________ (date).

**STG:** Resident will have increased attention span as is evidenced by sitting through ___________ (activity) for ___________ (number) of minutes, sitting through entire activity, ___________ (other) by ___________ (date).

**Problems/ Need:** Resident overtly occupied with self; with dressing; with eating; with the time of day; with name of ___________; with ___________ (other), etc.

**STG:** Resident will be able to remember the names of ___________ (number) of other people by ___________ (date).

**STG:** Resident will be able to discuss ___________ by ___________ (date).

**STG:** Resident will be able to locate clocks in nursing facility by ___________ (date).

**STG:**    Resident will be able to tell time by ___________ (date).

**STG:**    Resident will only change clothes __________ (number) of times daily by ___________ (date).

**STG:**    Resident will be able to remember ___________ by ___________ (date).

**Problems/ Need:**    Resident has difficulty making decisions; easily frustrated; overly dependent on others, etc.

**STG:**    Resident will be able to answer "yes" or "no" questions by ___________ (date).

**STG:**    Resident will be able to make a decision about sugar in coffee by ___________ (date).

**STG:**    Resident will be able to make a decision about ___________ by ___________ (date).

**STG:**    Resident will be able to locate ___________ by ___________ (date).

**STG:**    Resident will remain calm during decision making by ___________ (date).

**STG:**    Resident will be able to locate, remember ___________ without assistance by ___________ (date).

**Problems/ Need:**    Resident wanders around; needs constant supervision; often "scapegoated" by other residents; wanders into other residents' rooms; picks up items belonging to others; etc.

**STG:**    Resident will have appropriate outlet for excess energy as is evidenced by ___________ (only walking in approved areas, only walking in the hall, other) by ___________ (date).

**STG:**   Resident will only pick up items belonging to self by
__________ (date).

**STG:**   Resident will spend "wandering time" in group setting
with other residents by __________ (date).

**Problems/
Need:**   Unable/difficulty remembering others; difficulty identifying others; cannot remember names of __________;
exhibits fear when touched or approached by others;
etc.

**STG:**   Resident will be able to identify __________ by
__________ (date).

**STG:**   Resident will be able to remember name of ________
(activity director, nurses' assistant, wife, daughter, son,
other) by __________ (date).

**STG:**   Resident will be able to trust __________ (activity
director, nurse, nurses' assistant, volunteer, other resident, other) as is evidenced by not pulling away from
physical contact, not screaming when approached, not
striking out at other persons, other by __________
(date).

**STG:**   Resident will respond to ________ by __________
(date).

## Approaches:

1.   Use resident's name frequently during conversation, repeat
phrases as necessary.

2.   Gain resident's attention by speaking directly to him/her, maintain eye contact, stand or sit close to resident, speak slowly and
clearly using concrete terms.

3.   Allow resident time to respond; be patient and firm.

4.  Reward appropriate responses with smiles, nod of head, and verbal praise.

5.  One-on-one instruction on working with resident on (location of room, location of other); identification of __________; remembering __________.

6.  Ask "yes" or "no" type questions; allow time for response.

7.  Include resident in conversation regardless of response; do not talk about resident in his/her presence as if he/she were not there.

8.  Encourage resident to exercise choice, i.e., how coffee is prepared, in other; narrow choice to two or three items; do not hurry; allow resident time to choose.

9.  Do not scold resident during episodes of inappropriate behavior; offer gentle, but firm suggestions as to what is expected of resident.

10.  Assign resident volunteer, volunteer, staff, family member, other, to stay with resident during group activities.

11.  Assign volunteer, other to visit with resident to talk about events that occur in and around the nursing facility.

12.  Be observant of resident at all times, but do not restrain.

13.  Explain any activity before beginning; use repetition as necessary; be warm and friendly.

14.  During episodes of hostility or frustration, allow resident to express self. Help resident to identify feeling by making statements such as, "You sound angry," or "You sound upset...." Do not physically restrain unless resident attempts harm to self or others.

15.  Do not interfere when resident is arguing with another resident, but be observant to any physical contact that may occur.

16. Explain carefully to other residents to be more tolerant of this resident's behavior.

17. Be supportive of family; educate family as to resident's constantly changing behavior, encourage continued contact with resident.

18. Involve resident in the following activities:

a. _________ One-on-one for sensory stimulation to work on _________.

b. _________ Small group for sensory stimulation to work on _________.

c. _________ Current events discussion

d. _________ Nature walks

e. _________ Sing-a-longs

f. _________ Special exercise

g. _________ Special crafts

h. _________ Music listening

i. _________ Parties entertainments

j. _________ Other

# Amputation

Problems often associated with amputation include:

1.  poor self image;

2.  stump care;

3.  "phantom" pains;

4.  difficulty with ambulation, mobility;

5.  obesity;

6.  prone to pressure sores;

7.  difficulty transferring;

8.  needs assistance with ADL's;

9.  U. E. amputation — needs assistance with writing; needs assistance with feeding; needs self help devices evaluation;

10.  Prone to infection at surgical sites...

**Care Plan Information The Activity Director Could Use:**

**Problems/ Need:**  Poor self image; low self esteem; refuses to participate in group activities because of "the way I look...," etc.

**STG:**  Resident will be participate in group discussion for support and positive feelings about self and others by ___________ (date).

**STG:**  Resident will maintain positive self image as is evidenced by being up and dressed daily, participation in _______ (number) activities daily, other by __________ (date).

**STG:** Resident will be able to discuss feelings regarding amputation and self image with __________ (activity director, social worker, other) by __________ (date).

**Problems/ Need:** "Phantom" pains; complains of pain in amputated limb.

**STG:** Resident will use yoga breathing techniques daily to cope with pain by __________ (date).

**Problems/ Need:** Resident needs assistance writing; has difficulty writing; needs instruction for use of self help feeding device.

**STG:** Resident will be able to sign own name by __________ (date).

**STG:** Resident will be able to maintain own personal correspondence by __________ (date).

**STG:** Resident will be able to feed self by __________ (date).

**STG:** Resident will be able to feed with __________ (device) by __________ (date).

## Approaches:

1. Involve in group discussion with other residents who have similar problems.

2. One-on-one counseling with resident to discuss the origin of "phantom" pains; encourage resident to talk about the sensation and offer reassurance that "phantom" pains are a normal reaction.

3. Teach resident yoga breathing techniques as a means of coping with pain.

4. Obtain self help device and train resident to use.

5.  Involve resident in drawing classes to encourage use of remaining arm.

6.  Provide with paper and pencil; assist resident with daily writing exercises to gain control of use of remaining limb.

7.  Provide volunteer to assist resident with personal correspondence.

8.  Provide materials for self-learning experience to train in use of remaining limb.

9.  Include resident in the following activities:

    a.  __________ Sing-a-longs
    b.  __________ Parties
    c.  __________ Discussion groups
    d.  __________ Gardening
    e.  __________ Music
    f.  __________ Resident Council
    g.  __________ Religious services
    h.  __________ Entertainments
    i.  __________ Current events
    j.  __________ Pet therapy
    k.  __________ Exercise/movement
    l.  __________ Resident volunteer program
    m.  __________ Other
    n.  __________ Other

# Arthritis

Problems associated with the disease, arthritis, include:

1.  pain;

2.  diseased joints;

3.  bones break easily;

4.  fever;

5.  swelling of joints;

6.  pain on movement;

7.  increasing loss of mobility;

8.  limited movement;

9.  unable to ambulate;

10.  must be lifted for transfers;

11.  difficulty feeding self;

12.  difficulty writing;

13.  increasing loss of ability to care for self;

14.  needs assistance with activities of daily living;

15.  early morning stiffness; inability to move after prolonged periods of immobility;

16.  obesity;

17.  fatigue;

18.  anemia;

19. stomach, upper G.I., distress;

20. medication reaction;

21. weight loss;

22. poor self image;

23. needs motivation to do for self;

24. voices frequent somatic complaints;

25. excessive worry...

**Care Plan Information The Activity Director Could Use:**

**Problems/ Need:** Resident suffers swelling of joints; pain on movement; difficulty moving; increasing loss of mobility; early morning stiffness, inability to move after prolonged periods of immobility; etc.

**STG:** Resident will be participate in moderate exercise class daily by ___________ (date).

**STG:** Resident will participate in _________ (pottery class, bread baking, other) to exercise fingers and hands by ___________ (date).

**STG:** Resident will be able to do hand rolls __________ (number) minutes by ___________ (date).

**STG:** Resident will understand yoga breathing techniques as a method of coping with pain and will practice same by ___________ (date).

**Problems/ Need:** Resident has difficulty writing; inability to maintain own correspondence; wants to relearn how to write, etc.

**STG:** Resident will be able to __________ (write, print) own name by ___________ (date).

**STG:** Resident will be able to _________ (write, print) own correspondence by ___________ (date).

**STG:** Resident will practice writing __________ (number) minutes daily by ___________ (date).

**STG:** Resident will accept assistance of _________ (volunteer, staff) in keeping up with correspondence by ___________ (date).

**Problems/ Need:** Resident fatigues easily; unable to complete tasks because of fatigue; becomes tired on outings, etc.

**STG:** Resident will accept responsibility for own limits as is evidenced by resting for __________ (number) minutes __________ (number) times daily by ___________ (date).

**STG:** Resident will inform staff and/or volunteer when rest periods are required on outings by ___________ (date).

**Problems/ Need:** Resident has poor self image; low self esteem; refuses to participate in activities of nursing facility because of poor self image, etc.

**STG:** Resident will agree to discuss feelings with __________ (activity director, counselor) in _________ (feelings discussion group, other) by ___________ (date).

**STG:** Resident will participate in ________ (beauty shop, barber shop, good grooming, other) _________ (number) times weekly by ___________ (date).

**STG:** Resident will attend, participate in _____________ (activity) by ___________ (date).

**Problems/ Need:** Resident needs motivation to do for self; manipulates others to do for self those activities still able to do; is able, but not willing to ambulate, push own wheelchair, other, etc.

**STG:** Resident will be aware of manipulations and will ambulate _________ (number) feet assisted, unassisted daily by __________ (date).

**STG:** Resident will push own wheelchair _________ (number) feet daily by __________ (date).

**STG:** Resident will attend __________ (number) activities __________ (number) times weekly unassisted by __________ (date).

**Problems/ Need:** Resident voices frequent somatic complaints; uses somatic complaints as excuse not to participate in group activities; worries excessively about physical complaints, etc.

**STG:** Resident will participate in support discussion group by __________ (date).

**STG:** Resident will participate in _________ (activity) by __________ (date).

**STG:** Resident will agree to discuss feelings with __________ (activity director, counselor, other) by __________ (date).

## Approaches:

1. Involve resident in moderate exercise class for increased range of motion and mobility on S, M, T, W, Th, F, S (circle).

2. Monitor resident's participation in strenuous activities; use precaution.

3. Keep resident warm; avoid exposure to severe temperature; dress warmly.

4. Handle carefully when assisting resident to avoid pain.

5. Assist resident in regulating all activity to allow rest and avoid pain.

6. Provide resident with paper and pencil.

7. Include resident in activities such as drawing class, poetry class that fosters use of hands for writing.

8. Encourage resident to participate in pottery class for hand exercise.

9. Involve resident in bread making for hand exercise.

10. Instruct resident in use of yoga breathing techniques for control of pain; encourage use of same during acute episodes of pain.

11. Teach resident hand rolling exercises; encourage these to be done daily.

12. Evaluate resident for use of self-help devices.

13. Train resident for use of self-help device.

14. Involve resident in nutrition classes.

15. Counsel resident one-on-one about feelings.

16. Include resident in support group.

17. Verbally reward resident for tasks completed.

18. Encourage resident verbally to do for self.

19. Listen to resident's somatic complaints, but do not reward with question; report complaints to charge nurse.

20. Attempt to involve resident in following activities that allow for immediate gratification of good feelings about self:

a. ___________ Yoga breathing class
b. ___________ Moderate exercise class
c. ___________ Good grooming classes
d. ___________ Music discussion group
e. ___________ Beauty/barber shop
f. ___________ Other

21. Consult with family to avoid or lower stressful situations when possible.

22. Involve resident in the following group activities:

a. ___________ Resident Council
b. ___________ Parties
c. ___________ Entertainments
d. ___________ Exercise
e. ___________ Religious services
f. ___________ Movies
g. ___________ Cooking class
h. ___________ Committees
i. ___________ Bingo
j. ___________ Other
k. ___________ Other

23. Remind resident to shift weight and move around to avoid stiffness from being immobile during activities that do not require active physical participation.

# Cardiovascular Diseases, Congestive Heart Failure, Coronary Heart Disease

Problems associated with the diseases cardiovascular disease, congestive heart failure (CHF), and coronary heart disease may include:

1. edema;

2. hypertension;

3. excessive urination;

4. orthostatic hypotension, blood pressure fluctuations;

5. excessive confusion;

6. breathing difficulty;

7. shortness of breath;

8. coughing and wheezing;

9. cyanosis;

10. unable to participate in strenuous physical activity;

11. distress in limitation of activities;

12. exhaustion, fatigues easily, weakness;

13. insomnia;

14. medication reaction;

15. anorexia;

16. nausea and vomiting;

17. hypokolemia.

**Care Plan Information The Activity Director Could Use:**

**Problems/ Need:** Excessive confusion; unable to remember person, place, thing; difficulty identifying.

**STG:** Resident will be able to remember by ___________ (date).

**STG:** Resident will be able to identify ____________ by __________ (date).

**STG:** Resident will be able to locate ____________ by __________ (date).

**Problems/ Need:** Difficulty breathing; short of breath; unable to participate in strenuous physical activity; tires easily; exhibits distress with self in limitation of physical activities; use "weakness" as excuse not to participate in group activities, etc.

**STG:** Resident will practice breathing exercises ________ (number) times daily by __________ (date).

**STG:** Resident will increase tolerance to limited physical exercise to ________ (number) minutes daily by __________ (date).

**STG:** Resident will participate in moderate exercise class ________ (number) times weekly by __________ (date).

**STG:** Resident will take responsibility for self and rest________ (number) minutes, hours daily by __________ (date).

**STG:** Resident will participate in __________ (number) activities a week, month by __________ (date).

**Approaches:**

1. Include resident in awareness group.

2. One-on-one to remember ___________; to identify ___________; to locate ___________.

3. Include resident in daily discussion of current events.

4. Assign volunteer to visit with resident to discuss current events.

5. Evaluate resident for less strenuous activities; leisure counseling.

6. Encourage participation in activities that foster lung expansion such as sing-a-longs, yoga breathing classes, other, with physician's consent.

7. Encourage resident participation in activities that require a minimum of physical exertion such as bingo, parties, entertainments, other.

8. Involve resident in the following activities:

    a. ___________ Sing-a-long
    b. ___________ Current Events
    c. ___________ Discussion group
    d. ___________ Religious services
    e. ___________ Good grooming
    f. ___________ Movies
    g. ___________ Special crafts
    h. ___________ Music
    i. ___________ Beauty/barber shop
    j. ___________ Lecture series
    k. ___________ Cooking classes
    l. ___________ Moderate movement
    m. ___________ Moderate exercise
    n. ___________ Other

# Cerebral Vascular Accident Stroke

Problems often associated with the diagnosis cerebral vascular accident, or stroke often include:

1. paralysis (R) (L) side;

2. hemianethesia - loss of muscle joint sense, leans to one side;

3. mouth droops, excessive drooling;

4. difficulty swallowing;

5. muscle weakness;

6. fatigues easily;

7. prone to pressure sores;

8. loss of sensation of pain;

9. poor temperature control;

10. loss of bowel, bladder control;

11. incontinent;

12. difficulty writing;

13. difficulty with self feeding;

14. difficulty with ambulation;

15. needs (minimal, maximal) assistance with activities of daily living;

16. needs/using tube feeding;

17. Transient Ischemic (TIA's) attacks;

18.  seizures;

19.  excessive falling;

20.  elevated blood pressure;

21.  difficulty with vision;

22.  lacks peripheral vision;

23.  hemianopsia, only has vision on one side;

24.  aphasia (receptive, expressive);

25.  inability to formulate sentences; leaves words out;

26.  confuses words and visual images;

27.  unable to understand others;

28.  shouts out obscenities;

29.  inability to remember familiar names, places, numbers, people;

30   easily agitated;

31.  difficulty controlling emotions;

32.  involuntary crying;

33.  depression;

34.  disorientation;

35.  temporary amnesia.

**Care Plan Information The Activity Director Could Use:**

**Problems/
Need:** Paralysis (R) (L) side; difficulty writing; needs instruction for use of self-help device, etc.

**STG:** Resident will be print/write own name by ____________ (date).

**STG:** Resident will be able to pursue written communications with friends and/or family by ____________ (date).

**STG:** Resident will be able to feed self by ____________ (date).

**Problems/
Need:** Aphasia: receptive - unable to understand others, expressive - inability to formulate sentences; leaves words out; confuses words and visual images; shouts out obscenities, etc.

**STG:** Resident will be able to use _________ (communication board, flash cards, pictures, other) to communicate personal needs by ____________ (date).

**STG:** Resident will use written communication to express self by ____________ (date).

**STG:** Resident will verbally communicate with others in socially acceptable phrases by ____________ (date).

**Problems/
Need:** Inability to remember familiar names, places numbers, people; temporary amnesia following TIA's; disoriented, etc.

**STG:** Resident will be able to recognize name of _________ (roommate, staff, family, etc.) by ____________ (date).

**STG:** Resident will be able to locate _________ (room, activity room, dining room, etc.) by ____________ (date).

**STG:** Resident will be able to locate _________ (calendar, clock, etc.) by _________ (date).

**STG:**  Resident will be able to remember __________ (date, last meal, names of colors, etc.) by __________ (date).

**Problems/ Need:**  Easily agitated; depressed; cries easily; involuntary crying; poor self image; low self esteem; decreased interaction with others; etc.

**STG:**  Resident will agree to verbalize feelings instead of acting out by __________ (date).

**STG:**  Resident will participate in stroke group __________ (number) times weekly, monthly by __________ (date).

**STG:**  Resident will participate in __________ (activity) __________ (number) times weekly by __________ (date).

**STG:**  Resident will be out of room daily for __________ (number) hours by __________ (date).

## Approaches:

1.  Involve resident in writing exercises.

2.  Provide resident with pen and paper.

3.  Involve resident in activities that encourage use of hand and arm for writing such as drawing classes, poetry writing classes, other.

4.  Secure volunteer to assist resident with written communication.

5.  Secure self-help device and teach resident to use.

6.  Involve resident in feeding group.

7.  Provide pictures, communication board, flash cards designed to assist with personal needs communication; teach resident to use.

8.  Encourage participation in sing-a-longs and/or choral classes.

9. Use patience in talking with resident; allow time for response to conversation.

10. Counsel resident about language; let resident know it's okay to be frustrated, but not okay to curse.  Encourage other means of expressing frustration or bad feelings.

11. Take time talking with resident; explain slowly before each contact.

12. Use names frequently; identify self and others.

13. Involve resident in awareness type activities, such as discussion groups, current events, remember when, etc.

14. One-on-one with resident to work on recognizing __________, locating __________, and/or remembering __________.

15. Sensory stimulation to encourage awareness of surrounding.

16. Counsel with resident about feelings; help resident to name feelings and allow time for discussion.

17. Involve resident in activities that encourage physical release of frustration, anger, such as exercise, rhythm band, wheelchair volleyball, etc.

18. Involve resident in stroke support group.

19. Involve resident in activities that do not necessarily require use of both arms; encourage resident to exercise affected limb as much as possible.

20. Include resident in the following activities:

    a. __________ Sing-a-longs
    b. __________ Arts and crafts
    c. __________ Entertainments
    d. __________ Religious services

e.  __________ Music
f.  __________ Gardening
g.  __________ Resident Council
h.  __________ Beauty/barber shop
i.  __________ Parties
j.  __________ Exercise/movement
k.  __________ Pet therapy
l.  __________ Other
m.  __________ Other

# Closed Head Injuries

Problems often associated with people who have experienced closed head injuries include:

1.  inappropriate language; often curses; may make suggestive statement/statements with sexual overtones;

2.  limited or no impulse control; acts without thinking of the consequences;

3.  may express difficulty with authority figures; may "scapegoat" people in position of authority;

4.  problems with memory, both long-term and short-term; may not remember rules/policies;

5.  acts out feelings; may have inappropriate behavior; may act out sexual feelings;

6.  voice control problems; may speak very loudly;

7.  may have difficulty understanding abstract thoughts; may only be able to answer concrete questions;

8.  easily over stimulated; too many noises can over stimulate;

9.  likes to touch; can become aggressive;

10.  maybe very inactive; semi-comatose; comatose;

11.  may experience depression;

12.  may have difficulty with vision; hearing;

13.  may have low self-image; low self-esteem;

14.  may be much younger than majority of other residents;

15.  may need some assistance; total assistance with ADL.

**Care Plan Information The Activity Director Could Use:**

**Problems/ Need:** Resident uses inappropriate language, often curses during group activities and/or during one-on-one interactions with others.

**STG:** Resident will understand others do not enjoy being submitted to inappropriate language/cursing and will decrease to less than __________ (number) episodes per __________ (week, day, hour) by __________ (date).

**STG:** Resident will direct language into appropriate phrases such as __________ (give example of alternate phrase) by __________ (date).

**STG:** Resident will agree to discuss feelings behind the language with __________ (activity director, other) by __________ (date).

**Problems/ Need:** Resident makes suggestive statements/statements with sexual overtones.

**STG:** Resident will understand that others are not comfortable with open discussions or sexual innuendoes and will decrease behavior to less than __________ (number of times) each ______ (week, day) by ________ (date).

**STG:** Resident will take responsibility for his/her behavior, accept gentle reminders/confrontation, and stop inappropriate episodes immediately upon being reminded to do so.

**Problems/ Need:** Resident exhibits limited/no impulse control — often acts without thought to the consequences of his/her behavior.

**STG:** Resident will respond in positive manner to gentle reminders that his/her behavior is not acceptable in the nursing facility.

**STG:** Resident will increase number of appropriate interactions to ________ (number) _________ (times per day, week, month) by _________ (date).

**Problems/ Need:** Resident has difficulty interacting with people he/she perceives as authority figures; often "scapegoats" _________ (name, title of person: administrator, activity director, director of nursing, charge nurse, etc.).

**STG:** Resident will agree to discuss his/her feelings about _________ (name, title of person) with _________ (activity director, other) by _________ (date).

**STG:** Resident will agree to channel his/her negative feelings about ________ (name, title of person) into _________ (activity, be specific) by _________ (date).

**STG:** Resident will agree to explore feelings behind his/her anger for _________ (name, title of person) in ________ (discussion group) by _________ (date).

**Problems/ Need:** Resident has problems remembering _________ (rules, policies, time of day, schedule, ________ other), secondary to frontal lobe damage in brain.

**STG:** Resident will agree to participate in memory group _________ (times) weekly by _________ (date).

**STG:** Resident will respond to verbal cues of others and make appropriate choices _________ (1 of 5, 2 of 5, 3 of 5) _________ (number) times daily.

**STG:** Resident will be able to remember _________ (be specific) by _________ (date).

**Problems/ Need:** Resident has made sexual advances toward another ________ (male, female) resident.

**STG:** Resident will keep activity to private area over next 90 days.

**STG:** Decision of two consenting adults will be respected over next 90 days.

**STG:** Resident will respect the right of the __________ (male, female) resident to say "No" over next 90 days.

**STG:** Resident will agree to approach only those residents who are able to respond with consent over the next 90 days.

**Problems/ Need:** Resident grabs staff, other residents in sexual advances/ inappropriate manner.

**STG:** Resident will understand others do not wish to be touched by __________ (date).

**STG:** Resident's behavior will decrease to less than __________ (number) episodes per __________ (week, day) by __________ (date).

**STG:** Resident will find appropriate partner for his/her attention by __________ (date).

**Problems/ Need:** Resident has difficulty controlling sound of his/her voice; often speaks loudly.

**STG:** Resident will respond to verbal/visual cues to lower volume of voice as needed.

**Problems/ Need:** Resident has difficulty understanding abstract thoughts — is able to comprehend concrete language.

**STG:** Resident will be able to understand language of others by __________ (date).

**STG:** Resident will answer concrete questions correctly (1 of 5, 2 of 5, 3 of 5, 4 of 5, 5 of 5) by __________ (date).

**STG:** Resident will be able to communicate basic needs by __________ (date).

**STG:** Resident will interact with __________ (number) people per day by __________ (date).

**STG:** Resident will be able to express self as needed each day.

**Problems/ Need:** Difficulty making self understood; speech garbled and/ or disjointed.

**STG:** Resident will be able to communicate basic needs daily.

**STG:** Resident will be able to finish ________ (number) sentences (1 of 5, 2 of 5, etc.) by __________ (date).

**STG:** Resident will be able to communicate with others by __________ (date).

**Problems/ Need:** Resident is easily "over stimulated;" may exhibit inappropriate behavior when in crowded, noisy areas.

**STG:** Resident will respond to verbal/visual cues when his/ her behavior needs to be "put in check."

**STG:** Resident will take responsibility for self and move to quiet, less crowded area when feeling "overwhelmed."

**STG:** Resident will take frequent rest periods throughout day to avoid becoming "over stimulated."

**Problems/ Need:** Resident is semi-comatose; bedfast.

**STG:** Resident will respond to ________ by __________ (date).

**STG:** Resident will squeeze hand of activity director during one-on-one visits by __________ (date).

**STG:**  Resident will open eyes during one-on-one visits by ___________ (date).

**STG:**  Resident will look at activity director during one-on-one visits by ___________ (date).

**STG:**  Resident will ___________ (blink eyes, smile, other) during one-on-one visits by ___________ (date).

**STG:**  Resident will show signs that he/she enjoys ___________ (music, color flashing, other) by ___________ (smiling, slight change of coloration/flushing of skin tones, relaxing of shoulder muscles, other) by ___________ (date).

**Problems/ Need:**  Resident is experiencing poor self-image, low self-esteem; poor body image; depression; withdrawn from others; stays in room alone; refuses participation with others; decreased interaction with others; expresses suicidal thoughts, etc.

**STG:**  Resident will participate in ___________ (activity) ___________ (number) times ___________ (weekly, monthly) to build self-esteem.

**STG:**  Resident will participate in feelings discussion group ___________ (number) times ___________ (weekly, monthly) by ___________ (date).

**STG:**  Resident will agree to talk with ___________ (activity director, clergy, other) about negative feelings when contrary to personal health by ___________ (date).

**STG:**  Resident will spend ___________ (number) ___________ (minutes, hours) out of his/her room daily by ___________ (date).

**STG:**  Resident will agree to counseling with ___________ (person) by ___________ (date).

**Problems/ Need:** Difficulty coping with age difference between self and other residents; often sharp with other residents; impatient with residents who exhibit dementia, etc.

**STG:** Resident will visit with volunteer of same age group __________ (number) times __________ (week, monthly) by __________ (date).

**STG:** Resident will agree to discuss feelings of impatience with __________ (activity director, clergy, other) as needed.

**STG:** Resident will participate in discussion group with other residents to better understand their feelings __________ (number) times __________ (weekly, monthly) by __________ (date).

**STG:** Resident will be more accepting of other residents as is evidenced by more tolerant behavior when around residents exhibiting signs/behavior of dementia by __________ (date).

## Approaches:

1. Schedule visits with resident in private area __________ times a week.

2. Allow resident opportunities to talk about feelings. Be an active listener, make supportive comments such as, "I see what you mean" or "I hear what you're saying..."

3. Encourage resident to verbalize thoughts/feelings.

4. Encourage participation in discussion group as outlet for "restless" feelings, etc.

5. Encourage participation in exercise classes as outlet for restless, angry, sad feelings, __________ other.

6.   Provide therapeutic counseling, leisure education.

7.   Involve resident in feelings support group.  Motivate other residents to assert "peer pressure" as appropriate.

8.   When resident makes sexual advances, inform resident, "That's not why I'm here..." Do not scold. Gently remove resident's hand and walk away.

9.   Counsel with resident regarding privacy.

10.  Use gentle, verbal cues to remind resident of expected, appropriate behavior, language, _________ other.

11.  Inservice nursing staff regarding how to approach resident for care giving activities without sending inappropriate messages to resident.

12.  Inservice nursing staff on how best to communicate with resident.

13.  Do not joke or tease resident, resident does not understand joking/teasing.

14.  Take time to communicate with resident.  Use short simple phrases; repeat as needed.  Allow time for resident to respond.

15.  Mirror resident's speech; i.e., repeat back to resident what you have heard resident say.  Pay attention to gestures as well as phrases; attempt to understand.

16.  Encourage resident to interact with others, avoid isolation.

17.  Visit with resident one-on-one, provide support, help resident to identify feelings.

18.  Visit with resident for individual sensory stimulation program, work on _________ (name activity).

19.  Visit with resident one-on-one, monitor responses to visits. Talk about current events, activities of interest to resident such as _________ (be specific, based on resident's interest profile/ history).

20.  Provide volunteers to visit for socialization.

21.  Provide _________ (type of music, be specific) at bedside _________ (number) minutes each day.

22.  Read to resident at bedside from _________ (name book, magazine, etc. — be specific based on resident's interest profile/ history).

23.  Counsel with resident regarding behavior.  Let him/her know what is expected.

24.  Offer resident opportunities to discuss negative feelings about self; let resident know that these negative feelings are normal and part of the grief process.

25.  Allow resident to proceed through grief process at own speed; be supportive.  Provide counseling as necessary.

26.  Involve resident in discussion groups.

27.  Involve resident in activities that allow physical outlet for negative feelings, i.e.  wheelchair sports, crafts that involve pounding exercise.

28.  Involve resident in activities that do not put emphasis on the differences in physical functioning of participants, i.e.:

    a.  _________  Religious services
    b.  _________  Entertainments
    c.  _________  Casino nights
    d.  _________  Sing-a-longs
    e.  _________  Parties
    f.  _________  Music listening

g. _________ Movies
h. _________ Other

29. Secure volunteers with similar interests and of same relative age groups to visit with resident.

30. Encourage resident to maintain contact with friends/peer group by:

    a. _________ Assisting with phone calls
    b. _________ Offering place for privacy during visits
    c. _________ Assisting resident with correspondence
    d. _________ Providing transportation to _________ (place) for peer contact
    e. _________ Other)

31. Include resident in following activities:

    a. _________ Leisure education classes
    b. _________ Validation classes
    c. _________ Residents Council
    d. _________ Religious services
    e. _________ Cooking classes
    f. _________ Crafts
    g. _________ Exercise
    h. _________ Sports outings
    i. _________ Movies
    j. _________ Music entertainments
    k. _________ Discussion group
    l. _________ Other

# Diabetes Mellitus

Problems often associated with the disease diabetes mellitus include:

1.  elevated blood sugar;

2.  diabetic coma;

3.  insulin reaction;

4.  convulsions;

5.  frequent recurring infections;

6.  vaginal infections;

7.  gangrene;

8.  lesions of lower extremities;

9.  diabetic ulcers;

10.  decreased circulation;

11.  complications at injection sites;

12.  urinary incontinence;

13.  frequent urination;

14.  dry mouth;

15.  excessive intake of fluids;

16.  urinary tract infections;

17.  amputations;

18.  poor vision, blindness, retinitis;

19. loss of self image;

20. fear of complications of disease;

21. noncompliance with diet orders;

22. family interference with diet orders;

23. excessive hunger;

24. obesity.

**Care Plan Information The Activity Director Could Use:**

**Problems/ Need:** Decreased circulation; needs a daily program of exercise to promote better circulation; needs to be included in exercise class; etc.

**STG:** Resident will participate in exercise class _________ (number) times weekly by _________ (date).

**Problems/ Need:** Poor vision; blindness; unable to see clearly; needs to sit close to source of activity; vision blurred; etc.

**STG:** Resident will be able to locate areas of nursing facility without assistance by _________ (date).

**STG:** Resident will be able to locate activity areas unassisted by _________ (date).

**STG:** Resident will attend_________ (activity) by ___________ (date).

**STG:** Resident will attend _________ (number) activities by ___________ (date).

**STG:** Resident will sit close to source of activity at each coming by _________ (date).

**Problems/ Need:** Loss of self-image; low self-esteem; fear of further complications of disease; often depressed; spends much time in room; decreased opportunities for interaction and/or socialization with others; etc.

**STG:** Resident will be able to openly discuss fears as necessary by ____________ (date).

**STG:** Resident will be accepting of self-image as is evidenced by participation in group activities __________ (number) times ________ (daily, weekly, monthly) by ____________ (date).

**STG:** Resident will participate in group discussion by ____________ (date).

**STG:** Resident will agree to discuss fears with _________ (activity director, counselor, clergy, other) by ________ (date).

**STG:** Resident will spend ________ (number) minutes out of room __________ (number) times daily by ____________ (date).

**STG:** Resident will talk with __________ (number) other residents daily by ____________ (date).

**Problems/ Need:** Noncompliance with diet orders; eats from other residents' servings at parties; constantly snatching food away from other residents; buys food out of snack machine; "begs" for extra servings of refreshments at parties; etc.

**STG:** Resident will be knowledgeable about diet and consequences of noncompliance by ________ (date).

**STG:** Resident will take responsibility for own actions and stick with diet recommended by physician by ____________ (date).

**STG:**  Resident will agree to counseling with the dietitian by ____________ (date).

**STG:**  Resident will attend support group ________ (number) times weekly, monthly by ____________ (date).

**STG:**  Resident will respond positively to confrontation of staff and only buy those snacks that are allowed on physician's diet order by ________ (date).

**STG:**  Resident will agree to only consume those refreshments served to resident by ____________ (date).

## Approaches:

1. Include in group exercise each day; stress movement to promote increased circulation.

2. One-on-one to work on location of different areas of nursing facility.

3. Help to count steps from room to area of nursing facility.

4. During group activities encourage resident to sit in front or near source of leadership of activity.

5. When giving instruction, go slow; ask resident to repeat if necessary until instructions are understood.

6. Motivate resident to spend time out of room in company of others.

7. Counsel about self-image as necessary.

8. Let resident know if clothing needs adjusting or if color scheme can be improved.

9. Involve resident in support group discussions.

10. Do not tempt resident with non-allowed foods or refreshments.

11. Talk with resident before activity where foods might be served; let resident know what type of behavior is expected from him/her.

12. Monitor intake of refreshments during activities and report to food service supervisor and/or nursing.

13. Reward diet compliance with verbal praise.

14. Involve resident in the following activities:

   a. __________ Entertainments
   b. __________ Exercise/movements
   c. __________ Religious services
   d. __________ Resident Council
   e. __________ Grooming classes - for self-esteem
   f. __________ Manicures - for self-esteem
   g. __________ Adopted grandchild
   h. __________ Music
   i. __________ Parties - observe refreshment intake
   j. __________ Gardening
   k. __________ Beauty/barber shop
   l. __________ Volunteer visits
   m. __________ Volunteer visits
   n. __________ Resident volunteer program
   o. __________ Other
   p. __________ Other

# Gastro-Intestinal Diseases

Problems often associated with gastrointestinal diseases included:

1. nausea and vomiting;

2. diarrhea;

3. blood in stool;

4. pain;

5. stomach cramps;

6. unable to swallow;

7. gastrostomy;

8. colostomy;

9. chronic constipation;

10. weight loss, anorexia;

11. poor appetite;

12. depression;

13. mild confusion;

14. decreased involvement with others

15. occasional embarrassing episodes;

16. refuses participation with other residents because of somatic complaints, embarrassment, imaginary odors, other;

17. low self image.

## Care Plan Information The Activity Director Could Use:

**Problems/
Need:** Pain; etc.

    **STG:** Resident will use yoga breathing techniques to cope with pain by _____________ (date).

**Problems/
Need:** Depression; spends much time in room; limited interaction with others; low self-esteem; poor self-image; refuses participation because of somatic complaints, embarrassment, imaginary odors, other; needs to increase socialization with others; etc.

    **STG:** Resident will agree to discuss feelings with _________ (activity director, social worker, clergy, other) by _________ (date).

    **STG:** Resident will attend counseling sessions _________ (number) times _________ weekly by _________ (date).

    **STG:** Resident will increase time spent _________ (talking with others, sitting with others) _________ (number) minutes, hours daily by _________ (date).

    **STG:** Resident will have increased self-esteem as is evidenced by participation in _________ (beauty/barber shop, good grooming, other) _________ (number) times _________ (weekly, monthly) by _________ (date).

    **STG:** Resident will participate in _________ (number) activities _________ (number) times _________ (daily, weekly, monthly) by _________ (date).

**Problems/
Need:** Mild confusion; sometimes has difficulty (remembering, locating, identifying; decreased involvement with others, etc.

    **STG:** Resident will be able to locate _________ by (date).

**STG:** Resident will be able to remember ________ by __________ (date).

**STG:** Resident will be able to identify __________ by __________ (date).

**STG:** Resident will spend ________ (number) minutes, hours in social area daily by __________ (date).

**STG:** Resident will talk with _________ (number) others daily by ________ (date).

**STG:** Resident will attend ________ (activity) regularly by __________ (date).

## Approaches:

1. Educate resident as to yoga breathing techniques to cope with pain; encourage use of same.

2. Involve resident in discussion group with other residents.

3. Counsel with resident; provide opportunities to express feelings.

4. Involve resident in support discussion group.

5. One-on-one to discuss interaction with other residents.

6. Assign volunteer to visit with resident; friendly visits.

7. Encourage resident to spend time in social settings: living room, dining room, TV room, other.

8. Involve resident in beauty/barber shop, good grooming class, manicures, other.

9. Encourage resident to continue contact with family, friends, other.

10. One-on-one with resident to work on remembering ________.

11.  One-on-one with resident to work on locating __________.

12.  One-on-one with resident to work on identifying __________.

13.  Involve resident in daily discussions of current events.

14.  Involve resident in the following activities:

    a.  __________ Discussion group
    b.  __________ Resident Council
    c.  __________ Sing-a-longs
    d.  __________ Music
    e.  __________ Exercise
    f.  __________ Religious service
    g.  __________ Parties
    h.  __________ Entertainments
    i.  __________ Games, bingo, dominoes
    j.  __________ Nature walks
    k.  __________ Crafts
    l.  __________ Other

# Hypertension

Problems often associated with hypertension include:

1.   convulsions;

2.   dizziness;

3.   headaches;

4.   fatigue;

5.   insomnia;

6.   nose bleeds;

7.   blurred vision;

8.   shortness of breath;

9.   blindness or loss of vision;

10.  prone to heart attack and stroke;

11.  obesity;

12.  edema;

13.  medication reaction;

14.  hypokolemia;

15.  severe muscle cramps;

16.  loss of appetite;

17.  confusion;

18.  forgetful;

19.  inability to remember familiar names, places, people, things;

20.  loss of sexual drive;

21.  easily irritated;

22.  excessive nervousness;

23.  noncompliance with diet order.

**Care Plan Information The Activity Director Could Use:**

**Problems/ Need:**  Dizziness; fatigues easily; shortness of breath; etc.

    **STG:**  Resident will take responsibility for self and will rest _________ (number) times daily as needed.

    **STG:**  Resident will participate in activities that help to increase lung span, i.e., sing-a-longs, vocal exercise, other _________ (number) times weekly by ___________ (date).

**Problems/ Needs:**  Confusion; forgetful; inability to remember familiar names, places, things; etc.

    **STG:**  Resident will be able to identify _________ by ___________ (date).

    **STG:**  Resident will remember _________ by ___________ (date).

    **STG:**  Resident will be able to identify _________ by _________ (date).

    **STG:**  Resident will participate in current events discussion daily by _________ (date).

    **STG:**  Resident will participate in discussion group for current events by _________ (date).

**Problems/ Need:** Loss of sexual drive; complains of decrease in libido; easily irritated; excessive nervousness; etc.

**STG:** Resident will have positive feelings about self as is evidenced by participation in activities such as good grooming, beauty shop, other __________ (number) times __________ (weekly, monthly) by __________ (date).

**STG:** Resident will agree to discuss feelings as needed with __________ (activity director, social worker, clergy, doctor, other).

**STG:** Resident will participate in feelings discussion group __________ (number) time __________ (weekly, monthly) by __________ (date).

**Approaches:**

1. Observe for signs of distress when participating in activities.

2. Encourage resident to take rest periods throughout day.

3. Remind resident to rest for __________ (number) minutes in the a.m. and __________ (number) minutes in the p.m.

4. Involve resident in awareness activities.

5. Involve resident in discussion group with other residents who have similar problems.

6. One-on-one training to __________ (remember, identify, locate).

7. Counseling for acceptance of changes in behavior and desires.

8. Talk with resident daily about current events; encourage resident to participate in these conversations.

9. Encourage resident to continue contact with family, friends, other.

10.  Involve resident in the following activities:

a.  ___________  Moderate exercise
b.  ___________  Sing-a-longs
c.  ___________  Current events discussion group
d.  ___________  Games, cards, bingo, etc.
e.  ___________  Special crafts
f.  ___________  Entertainments
g.  ___________  Outside excursions
h.  ___________  Vocal exercise
i.  ___________  Feelings group
j.  ___________  Support group
k.  ___________  Music
l.  ___________  Resident Council
m.  ___________  Parties
n.  ___________  Gardening
o.  ___________  Other

# Liver Disorders

Problems often associated with disorders of the liver include:

1.  jaundice;

2.  itching;

3.  bruises easily;

4.  weight loss;

5.  malnutrition;

6.  nausea;

7.  excessive fatigue;

8.  accumulation of fluid in the abdomen;

9.  nose bleeds;

10. hypertension;

11. diarrhea;

12. dehydration;

13. medication reactions;

14. hepatic coma;

15. embarrassment;

16. depression;

17. low self-image;

18. fear.

## Care Plan Information The Activity Director Could Use:

**Problems/ Need:** Embarrassment; low self-image; concerned about what others may be thinking; refuses to participate in activities because of "looks," etc.

**STG:** Resident will learn to cope with embarrassment as is evidenced by participation in __________ (activity) __________ (number) times __________ (weekly, monthly) by __________ (date).

**STG:** Resident will participate activities that boost self-esteem such as beauty/barber shop, good grooming, other, __________ (number) times __________ weekly by __________ (date).

**STG:** Resident will agree to discuss feelings with __________ (activity director, social worker, clergy, other) __________ (number) times __________ (weekly, monthly) by __________ (date).

**STG:** Resident will participate in __________ (discussion, support) group __________ (number) times __________ (weekly, monthly) by __________ (date).

**Problems/ Need:** Fearful of consequences of disease process; expresses fear of dying; appears depressed much of time; withdrawn, stays in room; limited opportunities to interact with others.

**STG:** Resident will agree to discuss feelings with __________ (activity director, social worker, clergy, other) __________ (number) times __________ (weekly, monthly) by __________ (date).

**STG:** Resident will agree to counseling by __________ (date).

**STG:** Resident will agree to talk with __________ (number) of others daily by __________ (date).

**STG:** Resident will participate in __________ (discussion, support) group ________ (number) _________ times weekly by __________ (date).

**STG:** Resident will spend _________ (number) __________ (minutes, hours) out of room daily by ________ (date).

**STG:** Resident will participate in ________ (number) activities _________(daily, weekly, monthly) by _________ (date).

**Approaches:**

1. Avoid including resident in activities that may result in injury.

2. Check with dietary and/or nursing before serving any refreshments either liquid and/or solid.

3. Counsel with resident; provide opportunities to express feelings.

4. Involve resident in discussion group with other residents.

5. Involve resident in support discussion group.

6. Encourage resident to spend time in social setting; living room, dining room, TV room, other.

7. Involve resident in beauty/barber shop, good grooming, manicures, other.

8. Encourage resident to continue contact with family, friends, other.

9. Assign volunteer to visit with resident; friendly visitor.

10. Involve resident in the following activities.

    a. _________ Discussion group
    b. _________ Sing-a-longs
    c. _________ Exercise, moderate exercise

d. _________ Dances

e. _________ Entertainment

f. _________ Outings

g. _________ Nature walks

h. _________ Reading

i. _________ Resident Council

j. _________ Music

k. _________ Religious service

l. _________ Parties; check about refreshments before serving

m. _________ Games, bingo, cards, dominoes

n. _________ Crafts

o. _________ Movies

p. _________ Other

q. _________ Other

# Lung Diseases, Chronic Obstructive Pulmonary Disease, Bronchitis, Lung Cancer, Pneumonia

Problems often associated with diseases of the lung include:

1. short of breath;

2. fatigues easily;

3. needs $O^2$ in room prn;

4. insomnia;

5. cannot lie prone;

6. recurring respiratory infections;

7. cynosis;

8. prone to peptic ulcers;

9. episodes of acute respiratory failure;

10. chronic, excessive cough;

11. excessive secretions of mucous;

12. edema;

13. complains of pain on movement;

14. slow healing skin lesions;

15. obstructed airways;

16. tracheotomy care;

17. increased respiration/perspiration;

18. medication reactions;

19. loss of weight;

20. decreased appetite;

21. anemia;

22. fear of dying;

23. withdraws from others, stays in room;

24. spits on floor;

25. physical activities limited;

26. confusion;

27. frequent periods of depression.

**Care Plan Information The Activity Director Could Use:**

**Problems/ Need:** Shortness of breath; fatigues easily; limited physical activity; etc.

**STG:** Resident will participate in __________ (sing-a-long, vocal exercise, moderate exercise, other) __________ (number) times __________ weekly to increase lung span by __________ (date).

**STG:** Resident will take responsibility for self and rest __________ (number) daily as needed.

**STG:** Resident will participate in __________ (number) activities __________ (daily, weekly, monthly) by __________ (date).

**Problems/ Need:** Fear of dying; withdraws from others; spends much time in room; frequent periods of depression, etc.

**STG:** Resident will participate in group discussion for support and positive feelings about self and others __________ (number) times __________ (weekly, monthly) by __________ (date).

**STG:** Resident will spend __________ (number) __________ (minutes, hours) out of room daily by __________ (date).

**STG:** Resident will participate in __________ (number) activities __________ (number) times weekly by __________ (date).

**STG:** Resident will agree to counseling by __________ (date).

**STG:** Resident will talk with __________ (activity director, clergy, other) about feelings __________ (number) times weekly by __________ (date).

**STG:** Resident will go to beauty/barber shop __________ (number) times __________ (weekly, monthly) to increase self-esteem by __________ (date).

**Problems/ Need:** Resident spits on floor; throws tissues on floor, etc.

**STG:** Resident will use __________ (tissues, towel, spittoon) for spitting daily by __________ (date).

**STG:** Resident will throw tissues away in trash receptacles by __________ (date).

**Problems/ Need:** Confusion; forgetful about person, place, thing; has periods of inability to remember; short term memory is impaired.

**STG:** Resident will be able to remember __________ by __________ (date).

**STG:**  Resident will be able to identify __________ by __________ (date).

**STG:**  Resident will be able to locate __________ by __________ (date).

**STG:**  Resident will participate in discussion group for current events __________ (number) times __________ (weekly, monthly) by __________ (date).

**STG:**  Resident will discuss current events with __________ (activity director, other) daily by __________ (date).

**STG:**  Resident will participate in __________ (number) activities __________ (number) times __________ (weekly, monthly) by __________ (date).

## Approaches:

1.  Observe during activities, monitor for overexertion, shortness of breath, and other signs of distress.

2.  Include in yoga breathing exercise to maintain and/or increase lung capacity for air.

3.  Encourage frequent rest periods during daytime activities.

4.  During discussion type activities caution resident regarding over emotional types of outbursts.

5.  One-on-one counseling with resident about fears.

6.  Involve in group discussion with other residents who have similar problems.

7.  One-on-one training to remember, identify, locate __________.

8.  Encourage resident to arrange items in room in set places to avoid confusion.

9.   Encourage resident to sit in social area when watching TV.

10.  Encourage resident to spend time out of room daily.

11.  Invite and encourage resident to participate in:

    a.   __________ Bingo
    b.   __________ Moderate exercise
    c.   __________ Entertainments
    d.   __________ Crafts
    e.   __________ Resident Council
    f.   __________ Religious services
    g.   __________ Sing-a-longs
    h.   __________ Parties
    i.   __________ Sewing class
    j.   __________ Drawing class
    k.   __________ Discussion group
    l.   __________ Other
    m.   __________ Other
    n.   __________ Other

# Multiple Sclerosis

Problems often associated with the disease multiple sclerosis may include:

1.  difficulty with vision;

2.  speech sometimes slurred;

3.  increasing muscle weakness;

4.  muscles often spastic;

5.  spastic paraplegia;

6.  increasing loss of ability to care for self;

7.  needs assist with ADL's (partial, total);

8.  difficulty with self feeding;

9.  difficulty writing;

10. loss of bowel and/or bladder control;

11. nausea and vomiting;

12. prone to pressure sores;

13. difficulty breathing;

14. needs assist with transferring;

15. malnutrition;

16. decreased self-image;

17. fatigues easily;

18. becomes frustrated easily;

19. difficulty coping with emotional adjustment;

20. seems depressed much of time;

21. difficulty coping with age difference between self and other residents.

**Care Plan Information The Activity Director Could Use:**

**Problems/ Need:** Decreased self-image; low self-esteem; becomes frustrated easily; cries for no apparent reason; seems depressed much of time; difficulty coping with emotional adjustment; frequent mood swings; limited participation in activities because of emotional mood swings, etc.

**STG:** Resident will have basic understanding of disease process and its effects on emotions by _________ (date).

**STG:** Resident will participate in multiple sclerosis support group by __________ (date).

**STG:** Resident will have positive self image as is evidenced by participation _________ (number) times _________ (weekly, monthly) in _________ (good grooming, beauty/ barber shop, other) by __________ (date).

**STG:** Resident will verbalize feelings of ________ (frustration, agitation, hostility, other) as they occur.

**STG:** Resident will participate in __________ (number) activities _________ (number) times weekly by _________ (date).

**Problems/ Need:** Difficulty coping with age difference between self and other residents; often sharp with other residents, etc.

**STG:**  Resident will verbalize feelings in appropriate manner by _________ (date).

**STG:**  Resident will agree to discuss feelings with _________ (activity director, clergy, other) by _________ (date).

**STG:**  Resident will be more tolerant of other residents as is evidenced by _________ (friendly contact with other residents, lack of yelling at others, lack of sharp replies to the friendly advances of others, etc.) by _________ (date).

**STG:**  Resident will visit with _________ (number) others closer to own age by _________ (date).

**Approaches:**

1.  Allow time to talk and communicate needs.

2.  Do not scold or hurry resident

3.  Provide with self-help device and instruct resident on its use.

4.  Allow time to complete tasks; only assist as necessary.

5.  Use cheerful, matter-of-fact approach; avoid criticism.

6.  Offer opportunities to talk; encourage resident to verbalize feelings and/or fears.

7.  Involve resident in multiple sclerosis support group.

8.  Encourage participation in group discussion.

9.  One-on-one to help resident identify and verbalize feelings.

10.  Arrange for volunteer of resident's own age group to visit.

11.  Encourage continued contact with family and friends.

12. Assist in communication by dialing phone for resident, supply with paper and pencil for letter, provide volunteer to write letters for resident, (other).

13. Involve resident in activities that promote U.E. mobility such as drawing, writing classes, moderate exercise, poetry writing classes, other.

14. When resident is crying or appears depressed, offer assistance if needed or allow time to talk. Do not pressure for an explanation.

15. Educate resident to disease process; let resident know that mood swings are part of disease process.

16. Confront inappropriate behavior regarding other residents as such; let resident know what sort of behavior regarding other residents is expected.

17. Provide outlet for anger and/or frustration such as pottery, bread making, velcro darts, exercise, other.

18. Involve resident in activities that promote an increase in self esteem such as good grooming, beauty/barber shop, manicures, other.

19. Do not over-tire resident during activities.

20. Provide frequent rest periods during outside excursions.

21. Involve resident in the following activities:

    a. _________ Parties
    b. _________ Bingo, games, cards, dominoes
    c. _________ Discussion group
    d. _________ Current events
    e. _________ Crafts
    f. _________ Pottery class
    g. _________ Pet therapy
    h. _________ Movies

i.  __________ Entertainments
j.  __________ Religious services
k.  __________ Resident Council
l.  __________ Moderate exercise
m.  __________ Cooking class
n.  __________ Gardening
o.  __________ Friendly visitor
p.  __________ Other

# Parkinson's Syndrome

Problems often related with Parkinson's Syndrome disease may include:

1.  medication reaction;

2.  constipation;

3.  incontinence;

4.  increased perspiration;

5.  undue sensitivity to heat

6.  slow moving;

7.  postural gait;

8.  "cogwheel" motion;

9.  dyskinesia (muscle weakness);

10.  tremors;

11.  decreased ability to feed self;

12.  difficulty swallowing;

13.  difficulty writing;

14.  drooling;

15.  slow speech;

16.  flat affect;

17.  depression with mood swings;

18.  low self esteem;

19. easily agitated;

20. needs motivation to become involved with others;

21. decreased sexual functioning.

**Care Plan Information The Activity Director Could Use:**

**Problems/ Need:** Dyskinesia (muscle weakness); slow moving; fatigues easily; needs to participate in exercise to increase stamina, etc.

**STG:** Resident will participate in active exercise on (M, T, W, Th, F, S) by __________ (date).

**STG:** Resident will participate in yoga breathing exercise to increase lung expansion and stamina _________ (number) times weekly by __________ (date).

**STG:** Resident will take responsibility for self and rest __________ (number) minutes daily.

**Problems/ Needs:** Decreased ability to feed self, needs instruction for self help device; difficulty writing; difficulty ambulating wheelchair; increasing loss of control of U.E.'s, etc.

**STG:** Resident will be able to feed self with use of __________ (self help device) by __________ (date).

**STG:** Resident will be able to _________ (sign own name, print letters, notes, write letters, notes) by _________ (date).

**STG:** Resident will be able to ambulate wheelchair per self by __________ (date).

**STG:** Resident will participate in active exercise program to promote U.E. strengthening _________ (number) times weekly by _________ (date).

**Problems/ Needs:** Slow speech; frozen speech when upset; difficulty verbally expressing self; difficulty communicating personal needs, etc.

**STG:** Resident will be able to communicate needs daily by ___________ (date).

**STG:** Resident will learn to use yoga breathing techniques when upset to calm self and speak unhindered by _________ (date).

**STG:** Resident will read aloud for _________ (number) minutes daily by _________ (date).

**Problems/ Needs:** Flat affect; lacks muscle control of facial features; unable to smile, etc.

**STG:** Resident will participate in active exercise program per self to work on facial muscles ________ (number) minutes _________ (number) times daily by ___________ (date).

**STG:** Resident will be able to smile by ________ (date).

**Problems/ Needs:** Depression with mood swings; low self esteem; easily agitated; needs motivation to become involved with others; decreased sexual functioning; refuses to participate in activities with other residents, etc.

**STG:** Resident will have an increase in self esteem which is evidenced by continued participation in _________ (beauty/barber shop, good grooming, other) _________ (number) times _________ (weekly, monthly) by ___________ (date).

**STG:** Resident will agree to participate in counseling by ________ (date).

**STG:** Resident will participate in support group __________ (number) times __________ (weekly, monthly) by __________ (date).

**STG:** Resident will express self verbally in socially acceptable way when feeling agitated, depressed, etc. by __________ (date).

**STG:** Resident will participate in __________ (number) activities __________ (number) times weekly by __________ (date).

## Approaches:

1. Involve in active exercise program to promote muscle strengthening, stamina, U.E. strengthening, other.

2. Teach resident to use yoga breathing to maintain control of emotions during periods of frustration because of muscle tremors.

3. Involve in yoga breathing classes.

4. Encourage resident to rest for (number) minutes following periods of physical activity.

5. Obtain __________ (self-help device) and train for use.

6. One-on-one for writing exercises.

7. Provide paper and pencil for writing exercises per self.

8. Involve resident in activities that promote continued ability to write.

9. Allow ample time to express self verbally.

10. Encourage resident to continue to communicate verbally.

11. Encourage verbal reading exercises _____ (number) times daily.

12. Provide volunteer to talk with resident _________ (number) times weekly, daily.

13. Involve resident in activities that promote verbal communication such as sing-a-longs, discussion group, other.

14. Encourage resident to spend time out of room.

15. Involve resident in exercise class with emphasis on facial movement.

16. Teach resident facial exercise; encourage self exercise _________ (number) times daily for _________ (number) minutes; monitor progress.

17. Provide opportunities to talk about feelings.

18. One-on-one counseling to help resident verbalize feelings.

19. Involve resident in support discussion group with others.

20. Involve resident in following activities:

    a. _________ Exercise
    b. _________ Poetry Class
    c. _________ Parties
    d. _________ Games, bingo dominoes, cards
    e. _________ Religious services
    f. _________ Discussion group
    g. _________ Crafts
    h. _________ Resident Council
    i. _________ Movies
    j. _________ Cooking class
    k. _________ Entertainment
    l. _________ Current events
    m. _________ Newspaper
    n. _________ Sing-a-longs
    o. _________ Other
    p. _________ Other

# Peripheral Vascular Disease

Problems often associated with peripheral vascular disease include:

1.   poor circulation;

2.   stasis ulcers;

3.   gangrene;

4.   frequent blood clots;

5.   prone to thrombophlebitis;

6.   edema;

7.   pain;

8.   skin feels cool to touch, frequently complains of feeling cold;

9.   bluish and/or blanching appearance;

10.  cyanosis of lower extremities;

11.  skin becoming dry, taut, smooth, and hairless;

12.  poor self image;

13.  needs (maximal, minimal) assistance with ADL's;

14.  difficulty with ambulation;

15.  obesity.

**Care Plan Information The Activity Director Could Use:**

**Problems/**   Poor circulation; pain in lower extremities, etc.
  **Need:**

**STG:** Resident will participate in exercise on (M, T, W, Th, F, S, S) to promote increased circulation by _____________ (date).

**STG:** Resident will participate in yoga breathing class to learn to cope with pain __________ (number) times weekly by __________ (date).

**Problems/ Needs:** Poor self image; low self esteem; often makes statements such as "If only I had..." and "I just wish I could..."

**STG:** Resident will feel good about self as is evidenced by continued participation in events of nursing facility, i.e. will participate in ________ (number) activities _________ (number) times weekly by ___________ (date).

**Problems/ Needs:** Makes excuses not to participate in activities with others; spends much time alone in room; does not interact well with others, etc.

**STG:** Resident will have increased self esteem as is evidenced by participation in (beauty/barber shop, good grooming, other) __________ (number) times __________ (weekly, monthly) by ___________ (date).

**STG:** Resident will talk with _________ (number) others _________ (number) times daily by _________ (date).

**STG:** Resident will sit in social setting such as __________ (living room, dining room, TV room, other) for __________ (number) __________ (minutes, hours) daily by _________ (date).

**STG:** Resident will agree to counseling by _________ (date).

**STG:** Resident will participate in discussion group __________ (number) times __________ (weekly, monthly) by _________ (date).

**STG:**  Resident will participate in __________ (number) activities __________ (number) times weekly by __________ (date).

**Approaches:**

1.  Include in exercise class to increase circulation.

2.  Educate resident to avoid sitting with legs crossed or wearing of any garters or tight fitting clothes that would affect circulation; avoid positions which place pressure on extremities.

3.  Educate resident in use of yoga breathing exercise for coping with pain.

4.  Include in yoga breathing classes __________ (number) times weekly.

5.  Counsel with resident about disease process.

6.  Involve in good grooming, beauty/barber shop, and other activities that foster increased self esteem.

7.  One-on-one counseling to work on feelings.

8.  Involve resident in support discussion group.

9.  Encourage resident to spend time in social setting. Reward same with much verbal praise.

10.  Secure volunteer, friendly visitor to visit with resident.

11.  Visit with resident to chat about events in and around nursing facility.  Let resident know he/she is always welcome.

12.  Include resident in the following activities:

    a.  __________ Sing-a-longs
    b.  __________ Entertainments
    c.  __________ Music

|      |              |                             |
|------|--------------|-----------------------------|
| d.   | ___________  | Exercise/moderate movement  |
| e.   | ___________  | Resident Council            |
| f.   | ___________  | Yoga breathing class        |
| g.   | ___________  | Parties                     |
| h.   | ___________  | Movies                      |
| i.   | ___________  | Games, bingo, cards, dominoes |
| j.   | ___________  | Religious services          |
| k.   | ___________  | Current events              |
| l.   | ___________  | Crafts                      |
| m.   | ___________  | Other                       |
| n.   | ___________  | Other                       |

# Seizure And Epilepsy

Problems often associated with seizure and epilepsy may include:

1.  loss of consciousness;

2.  convulsion;

3.  need to watch for biting of tongue;

4.  prone to head injuries;

5.  falls frequently;

6.  confusion following seizures;

7.  memory loss following seizures;

8.  medication complications;

9.  stomach upset;

10. psychomotor attacks such as automatic purposeless movements.

**Care Plan Information The Activity Director Could Use:**

**Problems/ Need:** Confusion following seizures; memory loss following seizures, etc.

**STG:** Resident will be able to identify __________.

**STG:** Resident will be able to remember __________.

**STG:** Resident will be able to locate ________.

**STG:** Resident will remain quiet in bed following seizures until confusion/memory loss clears.

**Approaches:**

1. Observe for signs of warning prior to seizures.

2. Educate resident to be observant of warning signs so he/she may take precautionary measures and protect self from falling.

3. Observe for movement that appears purposeless; report to nurse.

4. Encourage resident to remain quiet following seizure activity.

5. Use resident's name frequently when talking with resident following seizure; give information regarding place, day, person, what has occurred.  Keep resident calm by using firm, quiet tones.

6. Do not involve resident in activities that cause undue stress and may trigger seizure activity.

7. Consult with nursing before involving resident in any activity that requires vigorous exercise or movement.

8. Involve resident in the following activities:

    a. __________ Sing-a-longs
    b. __________ Entertainments
    c. __________ Resident Council
    d. __________ Religious service
    e. __________ Discussion group
    f. __________ Music
    g. __________ Parties
    h. __________ Gardening
    i. __________ Crafts
    j. __________ Other

# Trauma To Spinal Cord

Problems often associated with spinal cord injuries may include:

1.    paralysis - paraplegia, quadriplegia;

2.    prone to pressure sores;

3.    prone to contractures;

4.    prone to (U.T.I.) urinary tract infections;

5.    neurogenic bladder;

6.    incontinence of bowels and bladder;

7.    needs assistance with ADL's

8.    poor temperature control;

9.    muscle spasms;

10.    needs assist with transfers;

11.    inadequate trunk control;

12.    manipulative of others; often demanding;

13.    personality adjustment;

14.    poor self image;

15.    depression;

16.    expresses suicidal thoughts;

17.    anorexia;

18.    obesity;

19.  difficulty coping with age difference between self and other residents.

**Care Plan Information The Activity Director Could Use:**

**Problems/ Need:**  Manipulative of others; often demanding; expresses much anger when desires are not immediately met; personality adjustment; curses, etc.

**STG:**  Resident will ask for wants/desires directly and not attempt to manipulate others by __________ (date).

**STG:**  Resident will be aware of the feelings of others and exhibit patience when requesting needs by __________ (date).

**STG:**  Resident will express feelings of anger, frustration through participation in __________ (crafts that allow much pounding, sports, exercise, other) __________ (number) times weekly by __________ (date).

**STG:**  Resident will participate in feelings group with other residents who have similar disabilities __________ (number) times weekly by __________ (date).

**STG:**  Resident will agree to counseling __________ (number) times __________ (weekly, monthly) by __________ (date).

**Problems/ Needs:**  Poor self image; low self esteem; poor body image; depression; withdrawn form others; stays in room by self; refuses participation with others; decreased interaction with others; expresses suicidal thoughts, etc.

**STG:**  Resident will participate in __________ (activity) __________ (number) times __________ (weekly, monthly) to help build self esteem by __________ (date).

**STG:**  Resident will participate in feelings discussion group
________ (number) times ________ (weekly, monthly)
by ________ (date).

**STG:**  Resident will agree to talk with ________ (activity
director, clergy, other) about negative feelings when
contrary to personal health by ________ (date).

**STG:**  Resident will spend ________ (number) ________
(minutes, hours) out of room daily by ________ (date).

**STG:**  Resident will agree to counseling with ________
(person) by ________ (date).

**Problems/**  Difficulty coping with age difference between self and
**Needs:**  other residents; often sharp with other residents; impatient with confused residents, etc.

**STG:**  Resident will visit with volunteer of same age group
________ (number) times ________ (weekly, monthly)
by ________ (date).

**STG:**  Resident will agree to discuss feelings of impatience
with ________ (activity director, clergy, other) as occurs.

**STG:**  Resident will participate in discussion group with other
residents to better understand their feelings ________
(number) times ________ (weekly, monthly) by
________ (date).

**STG:**  Resident will be more accepting of other residents as is
evidenced by more tolerant behavior when around
confused residents by ________ (date).

## Approaches:

1.  Confront manipulative behavior as such and encourage resident to ask for wants/desires directly.  Let resident know that other people get angry when they are being manipulated.

2.  Counsel with resident regarding behavior.  Let him/her know what is expected.

3.  Offer opportunity for resident to discuss negative feelings about self; let resident know this is part of normal process of grief for loss of self function.

4.  Allow resident to proceed through grief process at own speed; be supportive.  Provide counseling as necessary.

5.  Involve resident in group discussion.

6.  Involve resident in activities that allow physical outlet for negative feelings, i.e.:

    a.  __________ Wheelchair sports
    b.  __________ Crafts that involve pounding,
    c.  __________ Exercise
    d.  __________ Other

7.  Involve resident in activities that do not put emphasis on the differences in physical functioning of participants, i.e.:

    a.  __________ Religious services
    b.  __________ Entertainment
    c.  __________ Casino nights
    d.  __________ Sing-a-longs
    e.  __________ Parties
    f.  __________ Music listening
    g.  __________ Other
    h.  __________ Other

8. One-on-one counseling regarding identification of feelings; coping with same.

9. Secure volunteer with similar interests and of same relative age group to visit with resident.

10. Encourage resident to maintain contact with friends by:

   a. ___________ Assisting with phone calls
   b. ___________ Offering place for privacy during visits
   c. ___________ Assisting with correspondence
   d. ___________ Other

11. Encourage resident to spend time out of room; assist in ambulating wheelchair if necessary.

12. Counsel with resident regarding behavior with other residents. Explain the needs of the confused residents.  Let resident know that while he/she may not be able to hold a conversation with these residents, they do "pick up" on emotions expressed and negative behavior will only make them more confused.

13. Use behavior modification techniques, with physician's consent. Reward appropriate behavior with much verbal praise.  Ignore negative behavior.

14. Confront inappropriate behavior as such.  Let resident know what is expected of him/her.

# Urological Diseases
## Kidney, Urinary Tract Infections, Cancer, Renal Failure, Kidney Stones, Incontinence

Problems often associated with the different urological diseases may include:

1. uremia;

2. retention of urine;

3. foley;

4. supra pubic catheter;

5. recurrent urinary tract infections;

6. itching;

7. odor;

8. dryness of mouth;

9. pain;

10. bedrest;

11. incontinence;

12. loss of appetite;

13. weight loss, anorexia;

14. skin breakdown

15. medication reactions;

16. depression;

17. embarrassment;

18.  fear;

19.  low self image.

## Care Plan Information The Activity Director Could Use:

**Problems/**
**Need:**  Pain; itching; refuses to participate in activities because of somatic complaints, etc.

**STG:**  Resident will use yoga breathing techniques to control/cope with __________ (pain, itching) by __________ (date).

**STG:**  Resident will attend __________ (activity) __________ (number) times __________ (weekly, monthly) by __________ (date).

**STG:**  Resident will attend __________ (number) activities __________ (number) times __________ (weekly, monthly) by __________ (date).

**Problems/**
**Needs:**  Fear of dying; fear of illness, etc.

**STG:**  Resident will participate in support group __________ (number) __________ times __________ (weekly, monthly) by __________ (date).

**STG:**  Resident will agree to talk about "fears" with __________ (activity director, clergy, other) by __________ (date).

**Problems/**
**Needs:**  Embarrassment; resident expresses embarrassment over loss of control of bladder; low self image, depression; spends much time isolated in room; expresses anger using statements like, "Why me...," etc.

**STG:**  Resident will have increased self esteem as is evidenced by participation in __________ (beauty/barber shop, good grooming, discussion group, other) __________ number times __________ (weekly, monthly) by __________ (date).

**STG:** Resident will agree to talk about feelings with _________ (activity director, clergy, other) by _________ (date).

**STG:** Resident will be able to verbalize feelings with _________ (activity director, clergy, other) by _________ (date).

**STG:** Resident will participate in support group discussions _________ (number) times _________ (weekly, monthly) by _________ (date).

**STG:** Resident will spend _________ (number) _________ (minutes, hours) out of room daily by _________ (date).

**STG:** Resident will talk with _________ (number) others _________ (number) times _________ (daily, weekly) by _________ (date).

**STG:** Resident will participate in _________ (number) activities _________ (number) times _________ (weekly, monthly) by _________ (date).

## Approaches:

1. Educate resident as to yoga breathing techniques to cope with pain/itching; encourage use of same. Monitor progress.

2. Involve resident in yoga breathing classes.

3. Confront somatic complaints as such. Encourage participation in group activities.

4. Counsel with resident regarding feelings; be supportive of positive expressions, be empathic with expressions of fear, sadness, grief over self, etc.

5. Encourage continued grooming habits, makeup, hairdressing, etc. Provide resident with makeup.

6. Encourage participation in beauty/barber shop, good grooming classes, manicures, other.

7.  Involve resident in support group.

8.  Involve in discussion group with other residents.

9.  Assist as needed in making preparations for dying, i.e., contacting family members to say farewell, assist in making funeral arrangements, contacting clergy, other — as requested by resident.

10.  Encourage continued interaction with family, friends, other.

11.  Assist in making phone calls, writing letters, other.

12.  Provide volunteer to visit with resident; friendly visitor.

13.  Provide appropriate physical expression of frustration, fear, anger, other, such as exercise, crafts that involve pounding, other.

14.  Involve resident in the following activities:

    a.  __________ Crafts
    b.  __________ One-on-one visits
    c.  __________ Parties
    d.  __________ Resident Council
    e.  __________ Sing-a-longs
    f.  __________ Discussion group
    g.  __________ Religious service
    h.  __________ Exercise
    i.  __________ Supportive counseling
    j.  __________ Feelings discussion
    k.  __________ Entertainments
    l.  __________ Music
    m.  __________ Awareness Group
    n.  __________ Other
    o.  __________ Other

# SECTION III

## Glossary of Activities and Terms

# Glossary

An explanation of terms and activities suggested in the Activity Health Care Plan text.

**ADL** — Activities of Daily Living such as dressing, grooming, eating, etc.

**Abnormal lab values** — A term used to denote recent lab tests on urine, blood tissue, etc., are not normal or either high or low.

**Adopted family** — A volunteer person or family who has agreed to visit with a (perspective) resident on a regular basis.

**Adopted grandchild** — A child "volunteer" assigned to visit with a specific resident.  There is much information available through public library systems about beginning "Adopted Grandchildren Programs" in long-term care facilities.  Good sources of recruitment for these young volunteers include: youth programs at local churches, junior auxiliary of local VFW and/or American Legion, local grammar school classes, scouts, etc.

**Antidepressants** — Medication for depression.

**Antipsychotics** — Medication for people who experience total breaks with reality — psychotic episodes.

**Aphasia** — The result of an injury to that area of the brain that controls speech and/or speech perception; usually the result of a stroke or some sort of physical trauma; can be the result of a birth defect.

**Aphasia, expressive** — Residents with this type of aphasia often have difficulty speaking the words they have pictured in their mind; they may say "yes" when they actually mean "no."  While people who have expressive aphasia are not always able to speak, some are able to express themselves through the use of written communication.

**Aphasia, receptive**— Residents with this type of aphasia have much difficulty understanding the auditory symbols received from others, i.e., they are unable to understand the meaning of the words they hear.  Communication is extremely difficult for these residents because their understanding of language is all jumbled.  Communication boards and/or communication cards may be helpful.  These residents will respond positively to a calm, soothing tone of voice.  Expression of anger or frustration in talking with these residents will only produce frustration and anger on the part of the resident.  Patience and a warm, friendly attitude is the most productive mode of therapy.

**Approaches** — The statements of actions that others will take to help the resident achieve the stated short term goal.

**Awareness group** — A small group activity which develops or enhances the manner in which a person relates to himself, others, and the environment in which he lives. Preferably the group would consist of the leader and no more than five or six participants. Exercise could consist of:
1. role play situations;
2. discussion of feelings and/or opinions, or;
3. sensory observance situations.

**Auditory hallucinations** — Act of hearing that which others do not hear.

**Casino night** — A special event activity where a variety of games are set up for participants to choose from; i.e., poker, roulette, craps, black jack, etc.  Equipment can vary from the "real thing" borrowed from a local civic or social group who may use casino night as charity fund raisers or your own make shift equipment.

**Cognitive ability** — Ability to think and make decisions and remember.

**Cogwheel motion** — Act of moving around in a circular or repetitious position.

**Committees** — A group of residents who work together for a common goal.  Example:

1. newspaper committee - write a nursing home newspaper published (printed) weekly, monthly, or bimonthly;
2. decoration committee - make decorations for special events and/or holidays celebrated in the nursing facility;
3. refreshment committee - plan, prepare and serve refreshments for special events;
4. welcoming committee - greets new residents, orients them to nursing facility; or
5. entertainment committee - plans entertainments for special events, makes contacts, sets arrangements, etc.  (The list of committees is only as limited as your imagination and willingness to motivate others.)

**Communication board** — Pictures and words that represent the items pictured that enable people who are aphasic and/or otherwise have difficulty with language to express their basic needs to others.  Pictures and words may include that of a toilet, a hairbrush, a glass of water, a plate of food, etc.  These can be purchased through various companies that carry self-help devices; or they can be made by making simple line drawings or cutting basic pictures from magazines with the accompanying word symbol in bold print.  The resident is taught to point to the items which express his/her needs.  The boards can also be used to assist those residents who are able, to relearn speech.  The symbols should be large enough for the resident to see and point to effectively.  Also, it would probably be best to limit the number of symbols on each board.

**Cooking class** — An activity planned for residents to prepare a meal or some sort of edible refreshment.  If you are not fortunate enough to have a stove and/or some sort of kitchen for your residents to use, these activities can be planned and executed in the activity room in one of the following manners:

1. All food preparation up to the point of actual cooking takes place in the activity room; then the activity director takes the pots or baking pans to the nursing facility kitchen for use of the

stove or oven.  Then after it is cooked, bring the food items back to the activity room.
2.  Use portable equipment.  There are quite a few meals that can be prepared with just the use of a toaster-oven or a hot plate.

**Counsel: identify feelings** — Individual discussion with resident who is obviously acting out feelings.  For example:
1.  Resident is sitting alone looking out window crying quietly.  Activity director would identify feeling observed to resident and encourage resident to speak.  An opening comment could be, "Mrs. Smith, you look so very sad...?"  Pause and allow time for Mrs. Smith to respond.
2.  Resident is cursing at anyone who enters his line of vision.  Activity director could begin with, "Mr. Jones, you sound so very angry, what's going on...?"  Thus opening the door for Mr. Jones to talk about his anger and put an end to the acting out of his anger, and the cursing.  It is important to remember to allow the resident to speak his/her mind and not to moralize or otherwise grade the feeling as appropriate or inappropriate.

**Current events discussion group** — See discussion groups.

**Dance** — An activity planned for the purpose of moving with rhythm to music.

**Dementia** — State of confusion that may begin with memory loss and continue until all individuals' cognitive abilities are diminished or gone; a symptom of diseases that affects the brain or decreases the oxygen to the brain.

**Discussion groups** — An activity planned for the purpose of a verbal exchange of information between the participants.  Different types of discussion groups could include:
1.  Current events group - topics discussed are related to present happenings in the nursing facility, in the community, in the county, in the world.  Example: (a) prices at the supermarket; (b) planned special events in the nursing facility; (c) election of public officials; (d) unrest in the former Soviet block, etc.

2. Feelings discussion group - led by qualified volunteer or staff person for the purpose of examining emotions and learning to cope with these emotions.

3. Music listening discussion group - an activity planned for the purpose of listening to a variety of music types and discussing: (a) likes and dislikes regarding music played; (b) memories evoked by music played; (c) feelings evoked by music played, etc.

4. Remember when discussion group - discussion is provoked by a picture, an item, or an idea of events that occurred in the past. For example: (a) a washboard could be brought in by the leader and participants would be encouraged to verbalize how it was used, etc.; (b) a picture of a Ford Model T could be displayed for residents to discuss whether or not they ever owned one or rode in one, their favorite Model T stories, etc.; (c) at Christmas, or Easter, or Halloween residents could share their favorite holiday memories.  Remember when is only as limited as your imagination as a leader.

5. Support discussion group - led by a qualified volunteer or staff person for the purpose of reinforcing the participants' positive defense mechanisms through the use of encouragement, reassurance, advice, education, etc. Sources for volunteers to lead this sort of group could include: Muscular Dystrophy Association, Multiple Sclerosis Association, Alzheimer's and Related Diseases Association, Arthritis Association, clergy, MHMR, Department of Health, etc.

**Drawing class** — An activity planned for the purpose of allowing the participants to express their creative energies on paper with the use of pencils and/or charcoals.  Participants can draw from memory, from pictures posted, from still life set up for the purpose of sketching, from nature outdoors, from live models, etc. Beginners would work with basic shapes and learn to control their sketching medium.  Volunteers to lead this activity could include:

1. local high school art teachers or students;
2. teachers or students from local art schools;

3.  members of your local artist community; or
4.  craft store personnel, etc.

**Dyskinesia** — Act of impaired movement through space; inability of individual to relate where his body is in relationship to the environment exhibited by lack of balance or awkward jerking movement.

**Edema** — Swelling in the body caused by fluid retention.

**Exercise** — An activity planned for the purpose of self manipulation of muscle mass to preserve or regain health and mobility.  The different types of exercise recommended in this book include:

1.  Moderate exercise - primarily active range of motion whereby the participants stretch their limbs to the maximum extent possible. Example: head circles, leg circles and stretches, arm circles and stretches, etc.
2.  Movement - rhythmic manipulation of the body to music; often props such as scarves or rhythm sticks are used.
3.  Movement, moderate - as above with movement consisting primarily for the purpose of ROM not increased heart beat or pulse rate.
4.  Nature walks - ambulation out of doors along a specified route for the purpose of exercise and fresh air. This is a great activity to schedule early in the a.m. Just after or before breakfast or in the early evening just at sunset. Caution must be paid for those participants whose disease process or prescribed medications make them more susceptible to hypothermia or hypersensitive to the sun.
5.  Special exercise - movement and manipulation of the body designed specifically for those participants who are less able to follow directions than others, i.e. confused participants. This small group activity can best be done in a room that has limited stimuli so that the residents exercising are not easily distracted.  Special attention to good communication techniques by the leader are also helpful, i.e. use the residents' names frequently, be clear and concise in giving movement

instruction, circulate throughout the group physically assisting residents to move their limbs, etc.  Examples of instructions could include statements such as "Mary Jones, clap your hands; Linda Smith, kick your feet; Dolly Patterson, stretch your arms over your head; etc."

6.  Vocal exercise - an activity planned for the purpose of using the voice and expanding the lungs of the participants.  Singing out the alphabet, voicing rhythmic guttural sounds, reciting rhymes in a cadence are just a few of the fun exercises that can be done.

7.  Writing exercise - an activity planned to encourage and/or regain control in writing.  Repetition of basic shapes such as straight lines, curves, circles, continuous spirals, etc. are helpful.

8.  Yoga breathing exercise - an activity led by a qualified volunteer or staff member for the purpose of teaching relaxation and control over pain through the use of deep breathing.  Essentially the participants concentrate on the depth and extent of their breathing thus "shutting-out" the outside negative feelings and/or thoughts.  Sources for volunteers to lead this activity might include: a registered nurse (it is very similar to the Lamaze method of breathing for birth deliveries), the local YMCA or YWCA; local yoga training schools, etc.

**Entertainments** — Diversional activity planned for the pleasure of the participants who watch.  Examples:
1.  bands;
2.  variety shows;
3.  recitals; and
4.  dance exhibitions.

**Feelings group** — see discussion group.

**Flash cards** — Like communication boards, these are cards with line pictures and the word symbols for the pictures used for the purpose of communicating basic needs and/or relearning speech.  See communication board for more details.

**Flat effect** — Facial muscles are relaxed expressing no apparent feeling; not smiling not frowning.

**Good grooming class** — An activity planned for the purpose of enhancing and/or relearning basic hygiene. Depending on the level of the participants, exercise may include:
1. basic hand washing;
2. shaving;
3. hair brushing;
4. makeup and facials; and
5. manicures, etc.

**HCFA form** — MDS 2.0

**HCP** — Health Care Plan

**Hallucinations** — Act of seeing, hearing, or smelling what others do not.

**Hyperkinetic** — In constant motion, moving without rest.

**Incoherent speech** — Unintelligent speech; speech/speaking in sound; garbled.

**Incontinent** — Not able to control bladder and/or bowels.

**Insomnia** — Difficulty sleeping; having trouble sleeping.

**Lecture series** — An activity planned for the purpose of stimulating the intellect. The program planner or the activity director set up a program of speakers to talk and/or present slide shows on a variety of topics such as "Wildlife in Africa," "Fire Safety and You," "Love Poems of the Brownings," just to name a few.

**L.E.** — Lower extremities; legs and feet.

**Lethargic** — Display of limited or no obvious energy nor animation.

**Lip smacking** — Act of moving lips of mouth (making smacking sound); a symptom of tardive dyskinesia.

**Long term goals** — A long term goal is an overall statement of where the resident could be or what the resident will achieve over a period of time, usually a year of more.

**Long term memory** — Ability to remember events over an extended period of time, years.

**MDS** — Minimum Data Set is a minimal assessment of the resident.

**Manipulative** — Asking for wants or needs indirectly.

**Medicaid** — Title 19, financial aid for long term care residents; meets eligibility requirements.

**Medicare** — Title 18, financial aid/medical insurance for people over 65.

**Moderate exercise** — see exercise.

**Moderate movement** — see exercise.

**Mood swings** — Changes in outward expression of feelings; i.e. happy and laughing one moment, crying and sad, the next.

**Movement** — see exercise.

**Music listening** — see discussion groups.

**Nature walks** — see exercise.

**Neuro-muscular deterioration** — A wasting away of muscle tissue due to damage to the spinal cord or neurological system of the body.

**Newspaper** — an activity planned whereby the participants, write, reproduce, and distribute a communique (newspaper) regarding events and items of interest in the nursing facility to other residents, staff, and anyone who might enjoy reading it.  Articles could contain:

1. a welcome to new residents and/or staff with a brief biography of same.
2. happy birthday, residents and staff;
3. newsy stories about special events, parties, new activities, volunteers, etc.;
4. columns by the different department heads or their designees regarding "what's going on" in their area;
5. editorials;
6. sports information, etc.

**Nursing facility** — A health care facility duly licensed by the state, and which offers room, board, nursing care, and certain other therapies.

**One-on-one communicator** — See port-a-comm.

**OBRA** — The Omnibus Budget Reconciliation Act of 1987 also referred to as the Nursing Home Reform Act, that effected major changes in the operations of nursing facilities.

**Pet therapy** — An activity planned for the purpose of providing warmth and fun through contact with young animals such as puppies and kittens.  Sources for these unique volunteer visitors might include SPCA, local "zoo friends," staff's pets, volunteer's pets, your own, etc.  There is much information available about "pet therapy" programs at your local library. For articles on the topic look in the reference files.

**Phantom pains** — Physical sensation of pain, itching, etc. in an amputated limb.  Sometimes called phantom limb or phantom sensations; while the limb is missing, the pain and/or other feelings are very real.  This is a normal occurrence following an amputation.  It generally subsides or disappears over time.

**Port-a-Comm** — A device that can be purchased to enhance verbal communication with a person who is hard of hearing.  The device is battery operated and serves to amplify the speakers voice. There are a variety of these devices on the market.  This particular brand name is sold by Rhythm Band, Inc.

**Problems/Needs** — A problem is a situation or condition that causes or creates, or may cause or create distress for the resident; or interferes with the resident's adjustment or involvement with others.  A need is a condition which requires some sort of supply and/or relief.

**Prism glasses** — A self-help device used by people who do a lot of reading in bed and must either lay flat or have difficulty holding their book in the proper position.

**Prosthesis** — An artificial limb, breast, etc.

**R.O.** — Reality orientation.

**ROM** — Range of motion; extension and flexion of bone joints, limbs, etc.

**Rabbit trails** — Topics of conversation change from one noun to the next in the same conversation.

**Refreshment cart** — A portable rolling unit with coffee, juice, punch, and/or other snacks; served room to room usually by volunteers.

**Remember when** — see discussion groups.

**Resident Council** — A regularly scheduled discussion group whereby the residents who live in the nursing facility have an opportunity to voice their opinions regarding the operation of the facility, register complaints, and make suggestions.

**SOB** — Short of breath

**Scapegoated** — Act of placing blame for all the ills or what goes wrong on one person or thing.

**Self esteem** — How a person feels about himself.

**Self-help devices** — Instruments and/or equipment used to enhance independence in ADL; for example to achieve independence in eating one might use: plate guards, drinking straws, tippie cups, built-up handles for spoons, etc.

**Self image** — How a person sees himself; the visual image a person has of himself in his own mind.

**Sensory stimulation** — A series of progressive activities planned for the purpose of exciting or stimulating the senses; i.e. colorful pictures to stimulate vision, good smelling objects, to stimulate the sense of smell, different textured objects to stimulate the sense of touch, sounds to stimulate hearing, food items to stimulate the sense of taste.  Object: to stimulate the severely confused into being more aware of their environment, gain their attention and ultimately stimulate communication.  This can be done in small groups of two or three residents or on a one-to-one basis.

**Short term goals** — Short term goals are statements of action, on the part of the resident, that are behaviorally observable and can be measured over time.

**Short term memory** — The ability to remember or recall events which have occurred in the recent past, i.e. being able to remember what one has eaten for breakfast, etc.

**Somatic complaints** — The voicing of physical complaints or ailments.

**Special crafts** — An activity designed specifically for confused participants whereby they might experience the pleasure of expressing themselves through crafts.  Crafts used should be very simple by design such as finger painting, coloring, working with clay, cutting pictures, etc. As in special exercise, the groups should be small, two or three participants; instructions should be clear and concise.  Much patience and time should be allotted in planning special craft activities.

**Special exercise** — see exercise.

**Support group** — see discussion groups.

**Tactile senses** — Sense of touch.

**Talking book** — Books on cassette tape available at state libraries for the blind.

**Tardive dyskinesia** — Physical element/diagnoses which is a direct result of prolonged use of psychotropic medication.

**Task segmentation** — Act of giving information; in short simple steps — one step at a time.

**U.E.** — Upper extremities; arms.

**U.T.I.** — Urinary tract infections

**Universal cuff** — A device placed around the palm of the hand enabling the individual to hold a pen, pencil, brush, fork, etc.

**Universal sign language** — Gesture/facial expressions of thoughts or emotions.

**Urinary retention** — The act of the bladder holding urine.

**Validation Therapy** — A treatment approach to establish communication with residents who are not able to communicate through the use of language; residents who have decreased or lost communication skills.  This technique works on identifying the feelings behind the message from the resident and communicates to the resident empathy and understanding of the resident's feelings and the right to have these feelings.

**Vocal exercise** — see exercise.

**Volunteer** — A person who shares his/her time/talents, etc. without regard to being paid for these services.

**Wandering** — Act of walking or rolling a wheelchair aimlessly about without an obvious destination or goal in mind.

**Wheelchair volleyball** — A game of volleyball adapted for participants who are either in wheelchairs or sitting in a straight back chair. A net is set up separating the two teams. Participants are all seated (any number of people over six can play as long as the teams are evenly divided) and the "serve" is rotated from position to position; thus the participants remain stationary. The ball is either a nerf ball, a balloon, or a beach ball. Can be played indoors. Also known as "balloon volleyball."

**Withdrawn** — One who keeps to himself avoiding contact with others.

**Writing exercise** — See exercise.

**Yoga breathing exercise** — See exercise.

# Index

## A



## B

## C

Catheter 61
Changing awareness 25
Choice 107, 116
Choking 129
Circulation 230
Cognitive
  ability 25, 104
  pattern 27
  skills 55
Cogwheel 223
Colostomy 61
Combative 130
Communicate 72
  aphasic 48
  verbally 48
Communication 49, 79, 113
Complain
    32, 50, 65, 69, 73, 74, 129, 134, 153, 164, 200, 205
Comprehension 50
Confused 32
Confusion 131, 148, 174, 200, 204, 213, 233
Constant motion 33, 89, 131
Constipation 139, 141
Conversation 25, 69, 158
Crazy 72
Cries 25, 34, 78, 86, 153, 180
Curses 92, 152, 236

## D

Deaf 47
Decisions 34, 35
Decisions, difficulty with 57, 159
Dehydration 130
Demanding 236
Denture/bridge 129, 134

Dependent on others  159
Depressed  147, 180, 195, 200, 208, 212, 223, 236, 242
Derogatory comments  74
Dialysis  131
Diarrhea  65
Diet order  130, 195
Disorganized  108
Disoriented  148, 179
Disrobes  95
Disrupts  73
Distorted thinking  25
Distracted  25
Distress  104, 147, 174
Dizziness  139, 204
Dress  57, 130
Drooling  129, 223
Drowsiness  140
Dryness of mouth  129
Dyskinesia  224

## E

Edema  139, 203
Embarrassment  200, 208, 242
Expressive aphasia  48, 179

## F

Falls  127, 139
Falls asleep  25
Family  77, 130
Fatigue  169, 203, 224
Fear  36, 87, 147, 208, 212, 242
Feelings  77, 87
Fidgets  70
Flashes of light  41
Flat affect  87, 225
Forgetful  25, 129
Forgets  32, 33

# N

Needs
   assistance  43, 57, 59, 63, 163
   large print books  40
   talking book  43
   volunteer  43
Nervousness  205
Neuro-muscular deterioration  131
New resident  103, 118
Noises  50

# O

One-on-one  109, 148
One-on-one communicator  50
Overweight  137

# P

Paces  89
Pain  65, 111, 117, 129, 134, 164, 168, 200, 242
Participation  51, 104
Pressure sores  137, 141
Prosthesis  57, 127
Psychotropic medications  139

# Q

Quiet  96

# R

Rabbit trails  33
Rambles  49
Read  47
Read lips  47
Receptive  179
Receptive aphasia  48, 179
Recognize  31, 32, 41